A Woman's Guide
To Mental Health

by

Beryl W. Langley, M.D. and E. Joyce Stapp, M.D.

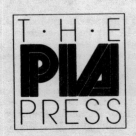

T·H·E
PIA
PRESS

This book is not intended to replace personal medical care and/or professional supervision; there is no substitute for the experience and information that your doctor or mental health professional can provide. Rather, it is our hope that this book will provide additional information to help people understand the changing role of women and the emotional and psychiatric problems that can evolve.

Proper treatment should always be tailored to the individual. If you read something in this book that seems to conflict with your doctor or mental health professional's instructions, contact him/her. There may be sound reasons for recommending treatment that may differ from the information presented in this book.

If you have any questions about any treatment in this book, please consult your doctor or mental health care professional.

In addition, the names and cases used in this book do not represent actual people, but are composite cases drawn from several sources.

The Facts About Jefferson Hospital

Your Center For Psychiatric Health Care

Jefferson Hospital provides psychiatric treatment in a calm, safe retreat-like setting for adults, adolescents and children who are unable to cope with the demands of everyday life due to emotional, behavioral, or substance abuse problems. Jefferson, a 100 bed private psychiatric hospital, is located on wooded acreage just minutes from all points in Louisville and southern Indiana. The setting of the hospital, as well as its design and furnishings, are specifically planned to foster a unique, therapeutic environment, meeting the diversified needs of patients and their families. Jefferson Hospital's dynamic, multidisciplinary team approach combines a variety of therapies to meet individualized patient treatment goals and provides opportunities for personal achievement as well as self-exploration. The physical needs of patients are met with a wide range of both indoor and outdoor activities. A confidence and trust building ROPES course provides a unique experience for many patients. Students can continue their studies without interruption through Jefferson's school program.

Free Assessments

Free consultations are available 7 days a week, 24 hours a day at the hospital or any of our convenient satellite crisis centers.

A trained mental health professional will talk over the problems you or your child is experiencing and will guide you to the level of care needed.

If you need our help, call 24 hours a day.

1-800-343-6722   **(812) 284-3400**

DEDICATION

To our families, for their love and support.

To the many women who have taught us to help others through their pain and struggles.

Acknowledgments

We are grateful to Marilyn Devroye, Dan Montopoli and Janet Chilnick, whose talents have been of great assistance in the organization and writing of this book. Our thanks also to Robert Stein, James Ledbetter, PhD and Ron Bernstein of PIA for their support and encouragement, and to Janice Lawson and Patricia Monroe of Jefferson Hospital for their assistance.

CONTENTS

Introduction: Why Women?

QUESTION: When we decided to write a book about mental health, why did we choose to write it about, and for, women?

ANSWER: Because medicine, by and large, still thinks of men as "the norm."

Following the normal training procedures, both of us graduated from medical school before going on to specialize in psychiatry. Throughout those years, as women, we experienced firsthand the male bias that runs through modern medicine.

Actually, we became uncomfortably aware of certain biases when still in high school. "Medical school?" friends of the family asked one of us in astonishment. "Why bother? A girl will never make it. Why don't you try nursing?"

Later, one of us was confronted by the family doctor, who had heard that his patient was applying to medical school; he issued a stern warning. "You'll never be accepted," he said, "and if you are, you'll never pass the examinations and if you do, you'll never get a job." (Some years after that, when his patient had successfully completed medical school, this doctor was the first one to offer her a job—in his own practice. She felt a certain glee in turning him down, explaining that she was going to specialize in psychiatry!)

When medical schools *did* accept us as students both of us experienced the same thing. Our families and even good friends fretted: "All that time and expense to become a doctor. You know you'll only give it up as soon as you get married and have children."

In medical school, some of the male professors (there were hardly any female professors) thought it was funny to slip a few female nudes into their slide presentations. To hide our anger and humiliation, we sometimes laughed along with the men students, or tried to. Getting through med school seemed to depend on being able to act like "one of the boys."

But it got much more serious than that. As medical students, we were taught to assume that men's symptoms were genuine, whereas women's symptoms might be largely "psychological"—in other words, unreal. Inwardly, we fought against this kind of discrimination. But outwardly, we still had to play by the rules. Many times, we found ourselves saying the equivalent of "yes, boss."

When we entered psychiatric training, we both found some sharp differences in the diagnosis and treatment of males versus females, but with no explanation for the discrepancies. Women had higher rates than men of major depression, agoraphobia, and simple phobia. Why? Compared to men, very few women were in treatment for alcoholism. Why? Almost two-thirds of all prescriptions for psychiatric medication were written for women. Why? There seemed to be no research in progress to help clarify these issues.

Worse yet, we began to realize that although pharmaceutical companies did extensive research on new kinds of medication, the subjects of their studies were most often men. As physicians, we knew that shifting levels of natural hormones could change the way a man's body would react to a medication. What about *women's* natural monthly hormonal changes, or birth control pills, or estrogen replacement therapy—how might these factors change dosage recommendations? There were simply no guidelines from the manufacturers of medications, so we concluded that no one knew.

More than ever, we were sure that our original conclusions had been correct: *Medicine, including psychiatry, traditionally discriminates against women, and a large part of this discrimination is unconscious.*

As we gained experience, both of us gradually came to realize that it's not just psychiatry or the medical profession. Despite some recent progress, our whole society in many ways still devalues women.

We came to realize that whenever we treated a woman patient, part of our job would be to find out how this automatic, usually unrecognized social devaluation of women was contributing to her problems. Her psychiatric treatment would be a learning process, as we discovered together how she could make changes that would revalue and empower her.

Over the years, we have seen many women psychiatric patients get better as they learned to reclaim and gain control over certain neglected, "lost" parts of their personalities. We rejoice whenever a woman tells us that we helped her make the shift from despair to hope, from helplessness to competence. And we have kept track of what works, so that we can use this knowledge to help other women patients.

We wrote this book to share some of what we have learned about women. We hope it will help patients, their families, and others to perceive that psychiatry can indeed change and grow. With insights gained from women themselves, psychiatrists *can* learn to recognize and respect the strength, energy, and potential of women—and help them in their quest for mental and emotional well-being.

1

The Invisible Woman

If you had to pick a single characteristic that most women share, what would it be? Attractiveness, seductiveness, intelligence, sensitivity, adaptability?

How about *powerlessness*?

Women come to psychiatrists for all sorts of reasons: for example, depression, anxiety, sexual problems, mood swings, or codependency on an alcoholic or drug-addicted partner. Sometimes the root of the problem is biological; depression and alcoholism, for example, are now known to run in families. Sometimes the root is social; too many children and not enough money are a stress-generating combination. In any case, whether women realize it or not, their lack of personal power and authority in the world contributes to their problems.

Often they *don't* realize it. That's because their powerlessness is part of a pro-male bias so deeply ingrained in our civilization that it goes unnoticed.

WHO'S IN CHARGE?

Think for a moment about who makes important decisions in the world. Most politicians, judges, and heads of corporations are men. Most journalists are men. Most doctors are men.

Then think about who carries out the orders of these decision-makers. Most low-level civil servants, paralegals, secretaries, research assistants, and nurses are women.

From childhood on, women learn in many subtle ways that this is really a man's world, and that they exist, and only *deserve* to exist, on the fringes. Even in an age of greatly expanding opportunities, the typical woman is terribly hesitant about developing her mind, spirit, and will. She still grows up believing she is defined by her ability to have children, and her willingness to support and nurture the men who really run the show. She senses that she can only share in the power structure by allying herself with a man who holds some of that power.

VIVE LA DIFFERENCE?

Any man who has read this far will be quick to point out that men love and cherish women precisely for their "differentness." But today, when the horizons for women are so much broader than they were in the past, women are asking themselves: Is it really an advantage to spend a whole lifetime as a cherished object—as someone who *is* rather than someone who *does*?

A girl may be brought up with as much education as a boy, but society still tells her that she's getting an education in order to be a wonderful wife and mother. Even though she may learn to admire independence, she is encouraged to value and encourage it in her sons and her husband—not necessarily in herself. This mind-set, which developed over thousands of years, is no longer functional in today's society. Unfortunately, however, it does linger on.

THE JOB OF WIFE AND MOTHER

No one lives in a cultural vacuum: all of us are shaped by the society we live in. As women emerge from girlhood, they gradually and naturally mold themselves to expectations that they will be nurturant, intuitive, and passive—i.e., "feminine." Without realizing it, they buy into the idea that they are, or should be, primarily child-bearers, child-rearers, and wives. For many women, becoming a mother does in fact lead to profound emotional growth and change.

But times have changed. Today, most people live in cities or suburbs and have relatively few children. Thus, mothering takes up fewer years of a woman's life than the past.

Ready-made clothing, electric appliances, and pre-pared foods have given us increased efficiency, but they haven't eliminated housework. Yet in modern American society, with its rich variety of lifestyles, the role of housekeeper is considered trivial. Particularly among younger women, there's a stigma attached to admitting that you're "just a housewife." What's more, the American economy has changed. Nowadays, it's the rare woman who has the luxury of being "just a housewife"!

A QUESTION OF FEMININITY

Despite smaller families, modern appliances, and a potentially wide choice of activities, many women are still caught in a cultural lag. Even today, if a woman decides that her primary identity is something other than wife-and-mother, she has to struggle with criticism that she is "unfeminine" or somehow unnatural, or that she is neglecting what should be her real role in life. Sometimes the objections come from men. Sometimes they come from women. Quite often the objections come from within, because the woman has internalized the idea that she can't really be happy unless she has a man and children to take care of.

For a woman, then, the overall picture is ambiguous. She sees that it's possible to develop certain characteristics that our culture values highly: independence, assertiveness, and personal responsibility. But she learns in more subtle ways that these characteristics are really not compatible with "femininity" —i.e., she'd better not develop them beyond a certain point, and certainly not to the detriment of her role as a nurturer.

COMING IN FROM THE COLD

Though bachelorhood may be some men's ideal, remaining a single woman often turns into a hard and lonely existence. A woman in America earns only 65 cents for every dollar a man makes, so she's economically disadvantaged right from the start. In addition, it's socially acceptable for men to do without women (i.e., in sports, clubs, or the military), but not nearly so acceptable for women to do without men.

If she follows the approved pattern of behavior, the single woman makes herself look as attractive as possible, gets a job, and then waits, hoping that some desirable man will eventually take her under his wing. This self-enforced passivity is the most demoralizing aspect of being a single-woman-searching-for-love.

In the classic scenario, attraction blossoms into love, and love leads to marriage. Babies arrive, and she quits her job. He provides the money; she provides meals, housekeeping, and child rearing; and they give each other emotional support and companionship.

In the old days, the ideal marriage was presumed to give a woman a house, children, and contentment. Today, however, the ideal marriage is expected to allow her something else: meaningful, paid work outside the home, *as long as it doesn't interfere with her nurturing responsibilities*. Usually her work turns out to be secondary to his; this is considered the price she pays for security.

WHAT GOES WRONG

But for many women, the marriage dream sours. If the husband is distant, condescending, or, worst of all, abusive, she suffers emotionally within the marriage. If he decides to leave her, she finds herself in trouble economically and socially—particularly if she's the one who keeps the children.

A marriage can go wrong in a million different ways. Here are some common stories:

- *He ignores her.* As children arrive, she focuses her energies on them while he spends more time and energy on his job. She cooks, cleans, and nurtures, but he doesn't notice or appreciate her efforts. They grow apart.

- *He dominates her.* Before they were married, he was courteous and deferential. Now, he treats her like the hired help. If she doesn't provide prompt service—such as meals and sex—he lashes out. He abuses her verbally or physically.
- *He belittles her.* His notions and his ideas are the only ones that count in their marriage. Since she's "only a woman" and doesn't work, her insights are of no consequence.
- *He expects her to be superwoman.* If she wants to go back to school or take a job, fine—but dinner had better be on time every night, and she'd better not neglect the kids, the laundry, home decorating, home repairs, bill paying, et cetera.
- *He beats her.* She's smaller and weaker than he, and he uses her as his whipping post whenever he's in a black mood. He roughs her up whenever he feels he isn't totally in charge of the household.
- *He doesn't provide for her and the kids.* The deal was that she would provide domestic services, and he would bring home money. But he doesn't uphold his end of the bargain. Alcohol and drug abuse may be part of the pattern in many of the stories.

Nevertheless, in many cases a woman stays married to a man she fears, hates, or simply dislikes. The reason may be emotional ambivalence, social pressure, economic necessity, or a combination of these.

THE "GOOD MARRIAGE"

Even in a "good marriage," the woman often finds herself playing a subordinate role. Most of us are culturally conditioned to assume that the husband is the main "doer" in the world, and that the wife's role is to take care of his physical, sexual, and emotional needs—as well as all of their children's needs. A "well adjusted" wife makes meals, keeps house, provides child care, and supports everyone else's projects. She may carve out her own niche of autonomy and individuality— *provided, of course, that she maintains her usual output of service to others.*

These assumptions about "what a woman ought to do" are a major part of our shared stereotypes about how life works. If a woman steps out of bounds by trying to get too much autonomy and individuality, or sheds part of her caretaker role in order to pursue her own dream of fulfillment, there will almost certainly be an outcry. And at least part of the outcry may come from within herself! Her husband and children aren't the only ones who think they're losing services to which they have a right; she probably thinks the same thing. In response, she may lash out in anger, or try to suppress her impulse toward autonomy, or vacillate between these two responses.

THE WOMEN'S PROGRAM

At Jefferson Hospital, we've organized what we call "the Women's Program," a therapeutic approach centered entirely on women psychiatric patients and their special needs. Through the years, we've discovered a core of problems that are common to *all* women in our society; therapy that addresses these problems forms the basis of our program.

In the Women's Program, patients get a great deal of education about the family as a system. They learn that the family is one of the great bastions of tradition in our male-oriented society, and that their own family may well work *against* them until certain changes are made.

Our women patients receive training in how to identify and express certain feelings, such as anger and rage, that they may have been repressing for many years. Plain old talk is very useful, and we've found several supplemental ways to help women express "stuffed" emotions:

- The *journal workshop,* which encourages them to write out their feelings.
- *Art therapy,* which encourages self-expression through drawing, painting, sculpture, or all three.
- The *quiet area,* for women who can center themselves through meditation or prayer.
- The *"angry room,"* equipped with foam-filled vinyl bags intended for beating and punching. Learning to express negative feelings seems easier for women in an all-women's group.

Probably the greatest triumph for our women patients is discovering that they have choices in life—that if they are caught in a vicious cycle of self-defeating behavior, they can break the cycle. This kind of learning happens best in a supportive group setting.

Patients grouped together quickly form a natural support system. Listening and talking to the other women, they learn from and reinforce one another in a way that isn't possible in mixed groups. They feel a growing sense of competence and self-direction, and they take real pleasure in accepting one another's strengths and weaknesses. This group learning reinforces and sustains the personal insights they are gaining in one-on-one therapy and gives them a chance to test what they have learned.

BECOMING VISIBLE

We saw earlier that women share the characteristic of powerlessness, and that the subordinate role is something they have been learning and practicing, unconsciously, since childhood. When a woman's recognition of her powerlessness begins to interfere with her ability to function, it's time for action. Must her happiness depend on finding and keeping the "right man"? Without a man at her side, or even with a man at her side, must she always be "invisible"?

The answer is *no*. A woman must become "visible" to feel emotionally healthy. In the following chapters, we'll see how psychiatry can help—or hinder—women's struggle toward first-class citizenship. We'll be focusing on how women can work to achieve autonomy and self-respect—in short, how they can *become visible* to themselves and others.

2

Traditional Psychiatry: Responsive to Women?

Although more women can now become doctors, most psychiatrists are still men. Psychiatrists, like everyone else, have absorbed the usual cultural standards, including the notion that women are passive and domestic while men are movers and shakers. Some psychiatrists may unconsciously assume that a woman's emotional or mental illness is less important, less significant, less *serious* than a man's.

WHAT IS MENTAL HEALTH?

Professionals don't like to admit it, but double standards do exist in medicine, including psychiatry. Often, doctors are unaware of the double standard. Back in 1970, however, the Broverman study showed this male-female split quite clearly.

Seventy-nine men and women who were mental health professionals—psychiatrists, psychologists, and

14

social workers—filled out a questionnaire about sex-role stereotypes. Each one received a list of 122 traits or types of behavior, such as:

very subjective ◄————————► very objective
not at all aggressive ◄————► very aggressive

They checked off which of these traits described healthy male behavior, healthy female behavior, and healthy (generic) adult behavior.

Result: The health professionals said a "healthy female" was less adventurous, less independent, less aggressive, less competitive, less objective, less interested in math and science, more submissive, more easily influenced, more emotional, more excitable over minor crises, more easily hurt, and more conceited about appearance than a "healthy male."

Most of them felt that the terms "healthy male" and "healthy adult" behavior meant essentially the same thing. This implied that *only men could enjoy complete mental health*! Women were in a no-win situation.

A BIT OF BOTH: ANDROGYNY

As women psychiatrists, we prefer the idea that *every* person has the potential for emotional and spiritual growth in many different directions. Even a "macho" man may have certain ladylike qualities, and a very feminine woman may have certain manly traits.

Think about it. Who hasn't met a couple where the wife has a good sense of direction, while the husband gets lost driving around the block? Or the wife scorns fashion, while the husband blow-dries his

> *"My husband, who is a career Army officer, likes to crochet. People think it's weird, but when he comes home at night what he does to relax is crochet while he's sitting in front of the TV. He did an afghan for every bed in the house, and now he's working on a wall rug."*

hair with mousse and a styling brush? Or the wife does the inviting, but the husband plans and cooks the meal? Math whizzes don't have to be boys, and the best babysitters aren't always girls.

> *"When we go on a family vacation, it's my wife who does the planning. She's the one who studies the map, figures out the times and distances, compares the rates at different inns and motels, and makes the reservations. She likes to do it, and frankly, I'm not that good at it. She has a lot more imagination for that kind of thing."*

A mixture of the masculine and the feminine in a person's personality is called *androgyny*. To our minds, androgyny is wholesome: it implies a balanced, highly developed character. The concept has been around for centuries; in fact, it's the basis for the ancient Chinese philosophy of Taoism.

In Taoist philosophy, the female and male principles are interdependent within a person—as symbolized by the above yin-yang illustration.

WHEN THE DOCTOR LIKES TO DOMINATE

Sigmund Freud believed that the psychiatrist/ patient relationship had to be one of superior to subordinate. No doubt some psychiatrists enjoy the feeling that they are their patients' parent, teacher, or savior, but this is usually *not* in the patients' best interest.

Sometimes a woman who feels helpless and dependent comes to feel she can't do without her strong, reassuring male psychiatrist, and the therapist encourages her to feel that way. When this happens, the psychiatrist/patient relationship embodies permanent inequality. It's a sad parody of sex stereotypes.

MISLEADING LABELS

The *Diagnostic and Statistical Manual of Mental Disorders, Third Edition, Revised* (known as *DSM-III-R*), published by the American Psychiatric Association, describes and names different psychiatric conditions. This manual gives psychiatrists and psychologists a common language for talking about their patients' problems. Often called the "Bible of psychiatry," the manual is nevertheless biased in some ways. Psychiatrists who rely on it too heavily may do women patients more harm than good.

Sex-Determined Diagnosis

One problem is that a woman may receive a different diagnosis than a man who has exactly the same symptoms. Take, for instance, "borderline personality disorder." *DSM-III-R* says that this condition, described as extreme instability in self-image, interpersonal relationships, and mood, occurs mostly in women. Yet this can work as a self-fulfilling prophecy.

Let's assume a man seeks psychiatric help because he is unstable in his self-image, relationships, and moods. Even though his symptoms sound just like those of "borderline personality disorder," the psychiatrist may rule out that diagnosis *because it's "uncommon in men."* The man may eventually be diagnosed as having "post-traumatic stress disorder" (PTSD), even though he had no particular trauma in his life.

So what's the harm? The danger is that borderline personality disorder is considered hard to treat, whereas PTSD is thought to be highly treatable. The "borderline" woman will face a doctor who thinks she's a difficult and perhaps hopeless case, whereas the "PTSD" man will deal with a doctor who thinks his problem is temporary and curable. Guess who will make more progress in therapy?

Sex-Biased Labels

Another problem with *DSM-III-R* is that its diagnostic categories may reinforce harmful sex stereotypes. Thanks to vigorous objections by psychiatrists concerned about women, three such categories have been deleted from the manual, but they do appear in the Appendix as "categories needing further study." They are:

1 *Late Luteal Phase Dysphoric Disorder,* formerly called "premenstrual dysphoric disorder." Since all healthy women menstruate, the existence of a diagnosis directly linked with menstruation could easily imply that *all* women had at least a touch of a mental disorder!

2 *Self-Defeating Personality Disorder,* formerly called

"masochistic personality disorder." This involves rejecting opportunities for pleasure, helping others while avoiding personal accomplishment, and sacrificing one's own interests. Objectors pointed out that these are features of traditional feminine behavior. Women learn them to gain approval and acceptance—and ultimately to get what they want. For women at least, this "disorder" is unfortunately the exact *opposite* of self-defeating behavior!

3 *Sadistic Personality Disorder,* involving cruel, demeaning, and aggressive behavior toward others. *DSM-III-R* says this problem is primarily seen in men. The trouble is that a rapist or wife-beater could attempt to be acquitted on grounds of insanity if a psychiatrist gave him this diagnosis.

DRUG-HAPPY DOCTORS

Therapists' attitudes toward their patients help determine what diagnoses are made and who gets treated how. Psychiatrists interested in women's problems worry that too often, "treatment" of a woman's mental or emotional problem amounts to medicating her, period. In other words, some doctors are quick to give women patients mood medication—not in addition to counseling, but *instead* of it.

Psychoactive medications have revolutionized psychiatry, but this revolution is a mixed blessing. Use and misuse of psychotropic (mood-changing) medication affects women's lives every day. Psychiatrists who are sensitive to women's needs have long suspected that women's reactions to mood-altering (and other) medications differ from men's. So far, however, drug companies aren't required to research the difference between women's and men's responses to various medications. The companies say they prefer *not* to study women, in fact, because women seem so complicated: their hormone levels vary throughout the menstrual cycle, they may be taking birth control pills, and so on. Of course, these are hollow excuses; a carefully designed study can overcome such obstacles.

Major Tranquilizers

The major tranquilizers (antipsychotics) help minimize "crazy" behavior, such as screaming, biting, scratching, kicking, and otherwise lashing out. Unfortunately, many seriously ill mental patients complain that the major tranquilizers dull their minds.

Doctors who aren't specially trained in the use of psychotropic medication may prescribe a major tranquilizer inappropriately. Many women patients who are given this kind of drug really need some form of antidepressant medication, plus counseling.

Some women who seem to have "major depression" really have a hormonal condition, such as thyroid deficiency. When the missing hormone is replaced, the depression lifts automatically. We can't overemphasize how important it is for the doctor to make a correct diagnosis before prescribing any treatment. Biologically trained psychiatrists use blood tests to help decide whether an emotional problem might be related to a physical condition.

Minor Tranquilizers

Valium and similar "minor tranquilizers" were originally thought to be harmless and were prescribed for anyone who appeared to be trying to cope with

> *"When I was seventeen I was very depressed, so my mother took me to a psychiatrist who put me on Thorazine. I now realize this was ridiculous: Thorazine is an antipsychotic medication, and I wasn't the least bit psychotic. I spent the whole summer feeling like I was looking at the world from behind a glass panel."*

stress. Over time it became clear that Valium for four months or more, at a dosage of 30 to 40 mg. per day, could lead to dependency and withdrawal symptoms very much like the symptoms the Valium was supposed to relieve.

Still, many people continue to take Valium, Librium, or Xanax month after month, and most of them—about 63 percent—are women. An estimated one to two million women are "hooked" on tranquilizers, alcohol, or a combination of the two, often with tragic results. Some 60 percent of drug-related admissions to emergency rooms involve women. More than two-thirds of these women have tried to commit suicide, often with a combination of Valium and alcohol.

Most prescriptions for minor tranquilizers are actually written by general practitioners, not psychiatrists. Many well-meaning family physicians are quick to prescribe a tranquilizer for a patient who complains of nervousness, tension, or anxiety. Our culture's tendency to encourage women (but not men) to adjust to passivity, weakness, and helplessness probably explains why more women than men are given tranquilizers.

"When I told my therapist that I would be moving to California because of my husband's job, he gave me prescriptions for Valium and sleeping pills 'in case I needed them.' Later, I realized I didn't need pills—I needed help in deciding to get out of my unhappy marriage."

Other Medications

Antidepressants can sometimes be a big help in relieving deep depression that doesn't seem to respond to "talk therapy" alone. Unfortunately, these medications are too often prescribed and taken willy-nilly.

Some antidepressants called MAO (monoamine oxidase) inhibitors can cause blood pressure to sky-rocket when certain foods are eaten, so the patient has to watch her diet carefully. Tricyclic antidepressants, which are chemically different from the MAO inhibitors, may cause dry mouth, constipation, and weight gain. Two fairly new antidepressants, Wellbutrin and Prozac, are less likely to cause such side effects. Often if a patient is not prepared for these side effects she will stop taking the medication on her own. The way in which these medicines are prescribed can minimize the side effects, but often general practitioners do not realize this, or in order to avoid the side effects, do not prescribe enough to relieve the depression. Also, these drugs are known to interact with other medications the patient may be taking.

Barbiturates such as Nembutal and Seconal, which may be prescribed for anxiety or sleeplessness, are more likely than the minor tranquilizers to cause overdose reactions and addiction. They are particularly dangerous in combination with alcohol.

Nonbarbiturate sleeping pills, such as Dalmane, Doriden, and Noludar, are also apt to cause adverse reactions and addiction, and are also dangerous when combined with alcohol.

SHOULD YOU TAKE PSYCHOTROPIC MEDICATION?

Women who are forewarned about overuse and misuse of psychotropic medication often wonder if the best policy is to refuse all mood-altering medication.

We feel that would be a mistake. For conditions that are basically biochemical disorders, medication may indeed be the most direct route to feeling better. If your energy level is so low that you can't even sit up straight, or if you can't help dwelling morbidly on your problems, you may need to take medication just to become receptive to psychotherapy. Medication can be a wonderful supplement to talk therapy.

However, because we do think a woman should be on her guard about mood-altering medicines, we offer these suggestions:

1 Be aware that not all doctors know how to prescribe psychotropic medications. In general, a psychiatrist is more skilled with these medications than a general practitioner.
2 If a doctor gives you a mood-altering medication, ask what it's supposed to do, how long you will take it, and what the risks are for getting "hooked." If you're not satisfied, ask for alternatives. If the

doctor won't give you any, consider finding a different doctor.

3 If you are uncomfortable with a diagnosis, don't be afraid to ask for a second opinion. Any reputable psychiatrist will be comfortable with this.

4 If your mood-altering medication doesn't seem to be working, or if it gives you side effects, make sure your doctor does something about it. The doctor might change the dosage, switch medications, or stop your medication altogether.

5 Insist on followup care. Don't assume that a prescription written six months ago is still right for you; you may no longer need medication. Remind your doctor that you are taking or have finished your medicine. At your checkup, ask if medication is still necessary. In many cases, the answer will be no.

6 Never stop taking a mood-altering medication on your own. With some products, it's essential to taper off gradually to avoid an unpleasant or even dangerous "withdrawal reaction" or relapse. Your doctor can tell you how to taper off properly.

3

What Are Little Girls Made Of?

Our culture treats girls differently from boys starting at Day One. If you doubt this, a trip to a newborn nursery will convince you. Newborn girls (dressed in pink for easy identification) are "tiny, sweet, and delicate"; newborn boys (conveniently dressed in blue) may be small, but are "hardy" and "game."

Of course, all newborn babies are relatively small and weak. What's at work here is a set of expectations about how the baby girl or boy will grow and develop. The ways we work to mark sex differences in infancy show that we still buy heavily into the traditional stereotypes.

As the infant grows, sex stereotyping continues. A mother lovingly fastens pink bows into hair no more than an inch long, to make sure everyone immediately identifies her baby as a girl. Pink booties and pink bassinet blankets are considered useless as hand-me-downs if the next baby turns out to be a boy.

Physical handling also differs according to the sex

of the child; most parents assume a girl needs gentler treatment than a boy. A father is apt to cuddle and stroke his daughter, but bounce and jostle his son; he believes the boy can take more roughhousing. Parents who think a slow walk around the block is sufficient exercise for a little girl may devote considerable time to teaching their small boy the rudimentary movements of baseball and football.

When a kid does step outside the sex-stereotype boundaries, many of us get uncomfortable. In preschool, for example, though the toys are available equally to all children, most teachers have certain expectations about who will use what. They may easily accept a little girl's enthusiasm for wheeled riding toys, but look askance at the small boy who spends a lot of time in the housekeeping corner. However, a girl's nonconformity in certain other areas is quite unacceptable; teachers and parents tend to find dirtiness or physical aggressiveness repulsive in a little girl, but more or less normal and tolerable in a boy.

Sex-role stereotypes are often counterproductive in today's world. Sometimes men need to be more nurturing, and women need to be be more assertive, in order to lead satisfying lives. Since the seeds of sexual stereotypes are sown in childhood, we need to be sensitive to the sex-role messages we give our children.

THE CARETAKER ROLE

Who takes care of baby? Usually it's the mother, at least at first. Biologically, she is the one who provides the milk (unless she chooses to give a bottle), so it's natural that she should have full charge of her baby in the early months. Full charge implies a lot of work; care of a small baby is a 24-hour job.

It's when she has small children that a woman is most likely to drop out of the paid work force. Since her husband is away all day at work, she assumes responsibility for all or most of the household chores. This creates the classic husband-at-work, wife-at-home scenario that many men find familiar and comforting. There's nothing wrong with this, except that the woman is likely to find it hard to break out of the caretaker role later on. Her husband and children have come to expect that she will provide them with many services—cooking, cleaning, laundry, chauffeuring, shopping—and what's more, she has come to think she owes them this. If she later decides to go to school or to work, she feels she has to squeeze in the new activity without reducing the services she provides. Her educational or professional activities seem marginal, to her and to everyone else.

It's important to realize that husbands, and children as they grow older, can and should learn to assume household responsibilities. There is no reason, other than custom, why the entire burden should fall on the mother. That just perpetuates the myth that a woman's place is exclusively in the home.

Naturally, single mothers don't have the luxury of coaxing their spouse to share in housework and child care. When their children are small, these women bear the crushing burden of full financial and caretaking responsibility. All the more reason why they should require that their growing children gradually take on a fair share of the housekeeping!

WOMEN: ROLE MODELS FOR GIRLS

As soon as a little girl realizes that she will grow up to be a woman, she begins to take cues from the woman she knows best. Typically, this is her mother. Eventually she perceives that housekeeping, which occupies a good deal of her mother's time, doesn't really count as work.

"Work" takes adults out of the home and puts them in contact with other adults. From the viewpoint of a small child in a traditional family, it's precisely because Daddy is away all day "at work" that he seems such a fresh, exciting visitor when he comes home in the evening. He swoops in at dinnertime with a joke or maybe a treat, then sits down to a meal he did not prepare. He relaxes in a living room he did not vacuum or dust, sleeps between sheets he did not launder, and breakfasts on food he did not buy. It's Mommy that supplies all these vital supports. Yet that is not what people call work.

Housekeeping wasn't always such a devalued task. Before the Industrial Revolution of the late 1800s, men ruled the world—from the father at home, through the village elders and the leaders of the church, to the statesmen who governed the nation—but women had skills that were essential to the survival of the human race. Women were definitely subordinate to men, but they were in no way helplessly dependent on them.

In Colonial America, for instance, married women had much more to do than sweep, dust, and take care of the children. Helped, if she was lucky, by her daughters and by female servants, a woman was expected to do all the following:

• plant the family's vegetable garden
• breed chickens

- care for cows
- make butter, cheese, and cream
- butcher animals for meat
- cook meals
- pickle and preserve foods for the winter
- brew large supplies of cider and beer
- card and spin wool
- weave, knit, sew, and mend
- make candles, soap, and herbal medicines
- heal common illnesses
- nurse the sick

The world depended heavily on women's work. Women literally had no time to question their role in life.

The social changes that accompanied the Industrial Revolution generated the so-called Woman Question: what would become of women in the modern world? Women and men have been wrestling with this question ever since. The answers, and lack of answers, continue to influence girls as they grow into women.

"RATIONALIST" AND "ROMANTIC" ANSWERS

One basic answer to the Woman Question was "rationalist": let women enter the marketplace as the equals of men. Let child rearing, cooking, and housekeeping become communal responsibilities, so that women too can be wage earners and thus achieve full equality. The trouble with this answer is the underlying assumption that the marketplace, the world of work, is a wonderland, an answer to all human problems.

The other basic answer to the Woman Question was "romantic": let home be considered a sacred temple of peace, and persuade women to continue to bask in domesticity. Women who felt constricted by the shrunken female role within the home might long to buy into the male dream, but the men who were living the dream knew it had a dark side. To many men, home—sweet, tranquil, noncompetitive—came to seem an absolutely necessary refuge from the inhumanity of the industrial world. And they felt that women, the traditional guardians of the hearth, were by their very nature the ones to keep the home fires burning.

The trouble with the romantic answer is that it ignores individual women's strengths and weaknesses. It assumes *all* women are intuitive, emotional, hopeless at rational thought, submissive, and self-effacing. In the romantic scheme of things, a woman ends up seeming a rather feeble-minded and silly creature.

DOCTORS AND STEREOTYPES

In the United States, the romantic answer largely won public opinion. Doctors and, later, psychiatrists enthusiastically promoted the idea that a woman's highest calling was to stay home and nurture men and children.

Even as more and more lifestyle choices opened up to women, the pressure to stay within the confines of a purely domestic role remained. In the 1950s and early 1960s, it was fashionable for a middle-class woman to get married right after high school or college and proceed to have four or five children. If endless domesticity proved boring, her doctor would be glad to prescribe pep pills or tranquilizers to mask her fatigue or depression.

In the late 1960s and 1970s, smaller families came into vogue. This caused women to ask themselves what, in addition to mothering, their role in life should be. All too often, doctors urged them to adapt themselves to the domestic role and not worry about finding a place for themselves in the "world of work." This advice proved dangerously shortsighted, since the rising divorce rate made single motherhood a reality for more and more women.

It was only during the 1980s—when the economy shifted so that most families needed a second income—that medicine in general, and psychiatry in particular, gradually got used to the idea that adult womanhood might encompass many roles, besides motherhood. Much work remains to be done; many psychiatrists still subscribe fully to the domestic ideal for women. But trails have been blazed. We are looking forward to the 1990s as a time of unprecedented growth in women's image of themselves—a time when women see themselves becoming visible in the world.

WHAT GIRLS WIN PRAISE FOR

Theories aside, our culture recognizes certain kinds of behavior as desirable for girls, and others as undesirable. These behavioral norms form the cultural backdrop for the typical girlhood. Let's look first at the so-called positive feminine attributes, and see how they can both form and deform a girl's personality.

- *Passivity.* Sitting still and paying attention, two of the hardest things for boys to learn in the early school years, seem to come easily to many girls. Yet passivity is not always an asset, and it can be a difficult habit to break later on. Many working women who know they aren't being paid enough find it impossible to speak up and ask their boss for a raise; the passivity that has become ingrained in their personality won't permit it.

- *Receptivity.* Listening to other people, responding to their feelings and wants, is a highly prized feminine characteristic that comes into full play during motherhood. In her relationships with men, however, a very receptive woman sometimes finds herself doing *all* the receiving. Ideally, receptivity should work two ways.

- *Submissiveness.* If she does what she's told, she's a "good girl." Yet beneath her submissive exterior, a girl who is subjected to unreasonable demands often seethes with resentment.

- *Self-deprecation.* Girls are encouraged to downplay and make light of their skills, since competitiveness isn't "feminine." Many girls habitually turn a compliment into an opportunity for self-criticism: "You really played well." "Oh, it was just dumb luck."

- *Sensitivity.* Tears and tender feelings are tolerated, even expected, in a girl. This is emotionally much healthier than the stoicism that's expected of boys. However, girls who dissolve into tears at the first hint of opposition or criticism are handicapped in their relations with other people, particularly in the workplace.

- *Emotionality.* Girls are expected to show their emotions rather freely. Although emotionality is liberating in principle, boys and men sometimes point to it as proof that girls' and women's volatility makes them unfit for work that requires self-control.

WHAT GIRLS GET DISAPPROVAL FOR

Now let's turn our attention to traits that are considered "unfeminine" and generally undesirable in a girl. It's interesting to note that in most cases these same traits are admired and appreciated in a boy.

- *Boisterousness.* By showing strong disapproval, parents tend to train their daughters out of rowdy, boisterous behavior. This makes the average girl somewhat more socially inhibited than the average boy.
- *Anger.* A girl is expected to show her anger indirectly—not by leaping up and punching the offender, but by sulking or crying. Eventually, this kind of training can make it hard for a girl to recognize her own anger.
- *Aggression.* Physical aggression against another child is strictly off limits for a girl. As a result, girls learn at an early age to be cruel and "catty" to one another rather than assaultive.
- *Competitiveness.* When a girl competes openly, whether for high marks in school, an athletic award, or a coveted job, people are likely to see this as a negative characteristic, a sign of ruthlessness.
- *Toughness.* It's considered somewhat unnatural for a girl to be tough and stoical. When punishment is meted out, a girl is supposed to show remorse and repentance, while a boy is expected to "take it" quietly and with little comment.
- *Insensitivity.* Lack of diplomacy—the tendency to ignore other people's feelings—is generally

considered less forgivable in a girl than in a
boy, since it clashes with the image of feminine
tenderness.

• *Feeling of entitlement.* A girl who walks into a
new situation fully expecting that people will
immediately like and respect her is apt to be
thought arrogant. It's expected that she will
show a certain amount of hesitancy and insecur-
ity—whether she feels it or not!

4

Growing Pains: Abuse of Girls and Women

Past or present abuse lies at the heart of what troubles many of the girls and women we see in our psychiatric practice. People commonly think of abuse as physical slapping or beating, but we are using this word in a much larger sense. To us, abuse is any sexual, physical or emotional mishandling that can cause lasting psychiatric damage.

"THEY WANTED A BOY"

"When I was a girl, I once brought home a math test to show my parents how well I had done: 95 percent. Their response was to point out that my older brother had got a 94 percent on his much harder *math test. I grew up knowing that no matter what I did or how well I did it, my brother would always be first in my parents' eyes, and I would always be second."*

Psychological abuse can be overt or, as in this case, covert. Parents who prefer sons to daughters may let their daughter know their feelings by failing to show her support and encouragement, or by actively discouraging and disparaging her.

Historically, and even in modern times, women have been under intense pressure to bear sons. Reza Pahlavi, the former Shah of Iran, once divorced his wife because she kept having girl babies instead of the male heir he required. In ancient China, unwanted female infants were often killed. Even today, some Orthodox Jewish men start each day with a traditional prayer thanking God that they were not born women.

In our "enlightened" society, the preference given to boy children is a cultural relic—supported by customs and traditions that seem innocent enough at first glance.

Traditionally, women who marry adopt their husband's last name. Many young women today keep their maiden name when they marry. But when they have a baby, what is the baby's last name—the mother's? the father's? If the child gets the mother's last name, does that imply that the husband isn't really the father? If the child gets the father's last name, isn't that just patriarchal? A hyphenated double last name seems unwieldy or somewhat pretentious. And when two people with double hyphenated last names marry, what last name should they give *their* children?

There seems to be no perfect answer to this sensitive issue. Some couples choose a new last name when they get married. This usually offends some of the relatives, but it certainly solves the "which last name?" problem when children are born.

Another custom is that most parents assume their

sons will have a career; unfortunately, too many parents still assume their daughters will get married, have children, and not need to work. This is a dangerous assumption because, as we pointed out earlier, the majority of American women need to work outside the home for an income, whether or not they get married and stay married. Telling a daughter she need not plan for a career is the modern equivalent of Chinese foot-binding. It not only perpetuates the notion that girls are economically useless or marginal, but also helps to keep women economically inferior.

We strongly favor training girls, as well as boys, for trades or careers, and we think it's crucial that women benefit from fair hiring and equitable promotion opportunities. Our modern, post-industrial economy can't afford to keep women on the margins of the workplace.

There is also a popular notion that a boy is an easy child to rear: rational, predictable, and steady. A girl is supposedly more difficult: emotional, capricious, and volatile.

It's time to raise our opinion of girl children's capacities and capabilities. Baby girls have a somewhat higher rate of survival than baby boys. Young girls tend to mature earlier than boys both mentally and physically. Teenage girls statistically have a far lower incidence of conduct and behavior problems than teenage boys.

SEXUAL ABUSE: A FAMILY AFFAIR

Cholly stood up and could see only her grayish panties, so sad and limp around her ankles. Again the hatred mixed with tenderness. The hatred would

*not let him pick her up, the tenderness forced him
to cover her. So when the child regained conscious-
ness, she was lying on the kitchen floor under a
heavy quilt, trying to connect the pain between her
legs with the face of her mother looming over
her.*—Toni Morrison, *The Bluest Eye*

Abuse can take the form of rape: a father, brother, uncle, or "friend of the family" may abuse a girl
sexually, particularly after drinking heavily.

Childhood rape is extraordinarily destructive to a
girl's developing emotions and sense of trust. Often
she tells no one, because she is ashamed and has no
words to describe what happened. Her mother may
know nothing about the rape—or perhaps she knows,
but feels powerless to do anything about it. The girl is
left with unexpressed and unresolved hatred and rage,
which gnaw at her from inside and can lead to depression, insomnia, weight loss or obesity, self-destructive
behavior, and suicidal impulses. Unfortunately, it may
be hard for a girl to convince other people that she
has been raped.

The emotional wound of rape heals badly, covered
by a weak scar that is likely to break open later in
life. A woman who was raped as a child will probably
fear or distrust her own sexuality; she may loathe
intercourse even with a man to whom she is drawn
emotionally. Rape by a trusted family member or
adult is even more destructive and confusing than
rape by a stranger. A child is taught to love and
respect her father/family yet rape doesn't feel loving.

During the 1980s, outspoken social workers lifted
the veil from family rape and began to educate doctors and teachers about recognizing sexual abuse in
children. Many hospitals are now equipped to help
child victims of rape. However, there is still plenty of
work to do in *preventing* the rape of children.

SHAMEFUL SECRETS

*"Daddy used to 'tuck me in' at night. I don't know
why my mother didn't check up on him—looking
back, I feel she should have suspected something,
because he took such a long time putting me to
bed. What he was doing to me made me feel
embarrassed and ashamed, but it never occurred
to me to tell anyone about it."*

Sexual molestation, another shameful secret that
often languishes in family closets, is a more subtle
form of damage than rape but just as scarring. Often the
girl whose father or brother molests her puts up with
it, even though it confuses and disturbs her, because
she craves the attention that goes along with it.

Our women patients who were molested as children
tend to think of sex as "something a man does to a
woman," rather than a way to express their own deep,
positive feelings. In self-defense, they learned in childhood to look upon sexual attentions with detachment.
This habit persists into adult life, interfering with their
ability to have a spontaneous physical relationship.

The problem is much more widespread than most
people assume: it's estimated that *one of every four
girls will be sexually abused before she reaches the age
of 18.*

Women who were sexually molested during childhood have a great deal to learn from one another as
they work their way out of the victim mentality, and
into sexual independence and spontaneity.

PHYSICAL ABUSE

*"My mother was always whipping me. She was
under constant financial and emotional strain,*

*because my father was an alcoholic who couldn't
keep a job. Looking back, I can see the pattern: he
would beat her, and she would beat me."*

Sadistic physical treatment of children does lasting emotional damage. There is about a 33 percent
probability that the physically abusing parent is an
alcohol or drug abuser. In some cases, however, as the
above quote shows, the alcoholic or drug-abusing parent physically abuses the other, codependent parent,
who then takes it out on the child.

Some women can trace their deep-seated feelings
of inferiority and worthlessness to beatings they received in childhood. Others have learned to fear men
because they grew up seeing their father knock their
mother around.

Physical abuse is habit-forming, and often gets passed
down from one generation to the next. Grown-ups who
were beaten as children are apt to beat their own children. Women and teenage girls, the ones who are most
likely to suffer beatings from men, may come to accept
physical violence as an inevitable part of family life.

A child who grows up in an atmosphere of physical abuse is certain to have emotional difficulties as
an adult. We recommend therapy for the whole family,
especially the abuser. If the child's safety can be
assured, it is better for the family unit to remain
intact. If safety is still an issue, the child should be
removed from the abusive environment.

ROLE MODELS FOR GIRLS

*"When I was a teenager, I could imagine gradu-
ating from high school and going to college and
traveling around the world and getting a job and
buying a car. In my mind's eye, I could see myself*

doing all those things. But when I thought about getting married, I could never get past the images of the wedding gown and the ceremony. When I tried to visualize my life after that, everything was dark. It was like having a black hole in my mind."

Historically, girls have been hurt by the lack of variety in female role models. According to the popular stereotype, reinforced by children's books, novels, and, later, television soaps and sitcoms, a girl's job was to grow up and be a housewife and mother. In this role she would be pleasant and competent, but rather uninteresting, because whatever she did would affect only her immediate family. She would mostly second her husband, helping him to advance in his career, applauding his successes.

Until very recently, "history" has really been "*his* story"—that is, the story of men and their achievements. Currently, feminist scholars are helping schools and colleges revise their curricula to reflect women's social contributions throughout history. For example, there have been successful women artists in all media for generations. However, they never commanded the same prices as their male counterparts and, until recently, were not mentioned in the standard textbooks.

Girls need to model themselves after other girls who strive, and women who succeed. They deserve to know that the child-rearing years are just one stage in what can be a varied, interesting, and productive life.

CHANGE COMES SLOWLY

Today there are several women role models in most fields; this means that girls have a better chance of developing their various potentials and abilities than their mothers had. Yet we still have a long way to go before girls of high intelligence and ability enter the professions in equal numbers with boys.

A few role models are not enough to erase the old stereotyped image of woman's place being in the home. Our country has woefully inadequate facilities for day care. Thus, for many women, having children still means dropping out of the work force. Many men, and even many women, still give professional women blatant or subtle put-downs for straying from domesticity.

In the office, the stereotypes die hard. A male boss may still expect a woman to make the coffee, no matter what job she holds. Some women employees still feel they have to work twice as hard as men to be considered "good."

Even when schools buy new gender-balanced textbooks, old cultural expectations still underlie much of what teachers think and say. Marjorie B. U'ren writes, "No one becomes a professional without encouragement; in a world that encourages few women to use their talents, it is inevitable that few women do so. Girls are not so much told that they cannot do something as *not* told that they can. And, if in spite of it all, a girl does decide to tackle a traditionally male profession, others are more likely to discourage her than to offer support."

Working mothers who find their work fulfilling are excellent role models for their daughters. The same goes for grandmothers, who from their long perspective are often more radical than mothers in their social outlook.

TEENAGE GIRLS' SOCIAL CRISES

"When I got my first period, my parents were sitting outside on the patio with some guests. I

called out the window and asked my mother if she could come upstairs for a minute. And of course all the guests figured out right away what was happening. I was so embarrassed I could have died."

"This whole high school runs on a system of cliques. Only a few people aren't in any clique at all, and they are really out of it. They just have no social life, period."

As a girl moves into her teens, she is buffeted by increasingly high waves of physical change and social pressure:

- *Menstruation* signals the start of her potential reproductive life, and with it comes worries about body image, sex, pregnancy, and contraception.
- *Hormonal changes* that accompany menstruation may expand her range of moods and emotions, surprising and confusing her at first.
- *Popularity* at school becomes a top priority; she dresses, talks, eats, and buys with an eye to impressing certain other teens with her good taste.
- *Acting feminine* may mean giving up certain formerly cherished activities and clothes: sandlot baseball and grass-stained jeans give way to modelling classes and designer-look outfits.
- *Dating* looms as an intimidating possibility, raising several questions: How do I attract a boy? How do I act when we're together? How physical should we get?
- *Competing* for boys' interest and attention may strain her relationships with other girls.

The teen years are inherently tension-filled as horizons expand and personal responsibilities increase. Certain psychiatric patterns emerge among teenage girls who find the tensions overwhelming. Heading the list are alcohol and drug abuse, depression, eating disorders, and suicide attempts.

Parents who delay seeking competent help for their emotionally troubled daughter are probably making a mistake. We find that for virtually any psychiatric problem, early treatment works faster and better than late treatment.

EXPECTATIONS ABOUT MONEY

It is largely during adolescence that girls form their attitude toward money. Our culture sends girls a disturbing double message.

1 Women have money and enormous economic power. Since they are the ones who do most of their family's shopping, they actually control most of the wealth of this country.
2 Women know nothing about money and power, nor do they care to know; they do not have "a head for business."

There is a further message girls perceive through various cultural cues: A "real lady," the most elegant kind of woman there is, does not have to work to earn money; as the daughter of a wealthy man, she comes "already paid for." This myth, so widely accepted that it's virtually invisible to most people, helps explain why most women deny that keeping house, cooking meals, or rearing children is work.

Parents should make sure their daughters know the facts behind the myths:

1 Women do *not* control the wealth of America. Most investments are carried out by institutions, which are largely controlled by men, and most consumer products are conceived, designed, and marketed by men.
2 For much of Western history, women were confined to the home, where they remained totally ignorant of the world of business. Given an equal chance, however, women can have as much of a "head for business" as men. Business acumen is learned, not inborn.
3 Keeping a household is most definitely work, the more so if there are children. Ask any man who has had to take care of the house and kids while his wife was away! Our very civilization depends on the largely unacknowledged and only indirectly "paid" labor of wives and mothers.

Keeping women ignorant about money is a form of social abuse. In order to assume an economically responsible place in society, a girl needs to learn the basics of finance. Parents should make sure their teenage daughter learns how to open a bank account, balance a checkbook, obtain credit, make and stick to a budget, invest money, and follow her investments intelligently. If money is power, and if women hope to acquire more power over their lives—to emerge from invisibility—they need to be on familiar terms with the management of money.

In our practice, we strive to help women and teenage girls deal with those aspects of survival—planning, making life decisions, earning money—that they formerly may have left to their father, boyfriend, or husband. As a woman learns to control these forces, she gains psychological strength. Gradually, she becomes more visible to others and, most importantly, to herself.

5

Bad Girls: Delinquency and Promiscuity

Some of our young patients have been brought to the hospital because they are "out of control"—delinquent and promiscuous. It's fair enough to search for the reasons and to show them how they might change, if only because such behavior can endanger their lives. But first we'd like to discuss the psychological infrastructure of delinquency and promiscuity.

SEXUAL CONFORMITY

In America today, the stereotype of the "lady" —cool, elegant, and passive—is still alive and well. For some girls and women, this stereotype seems as easy to slip into as a tailor-made garment. For others, who are more active and reckless, the stereotype fits like a cultural straitjacket. To preserve their personal identity, these women need to rebel.

Everyone likes approval. Then why do some people deliberately act in ways that brand them as wild, unmanageable, and dangerous? Usually it's because they are not what society tells them they should be, and they can't see how to resolve these differences constructively.

Because of anger, low self-esteem, or both, the "bad girl" has decided that she can't or won't compete for prizes and praise. Instead, she opts to get what she wants, and damn the consequences. She makes do with what's called *negative attention*—reproach and, sometimes, punishment. She gets stimulation through delinquency.

Several kinds of behavior qualify as delinquent:

- not showing up for school or work
- bad-mouthing a parent, a teacher, the boss, or some other authority figure
- ignoring family curfews; staying out late or all night
- smoking and drinking when she is underage, or at forbidden times and places
- using and/or dealing illegal drugs
- shoplifting
- dressing provocatively in clothes that are tight-fitting, low-cut, or too sheer
- using exaggerated make-up
- trading sexual favors for drugs or money

Achievement and delinquency are not mutually exclusive. A high achiever may ace her chemistry course, but get arrested for shoplifting. She may star on the basketball team, but get thrown out of home economics for sassing the teacher.

Parents are usually very concerned about a delinquent daughter. They worry that she will get pregnant, or be expelled from school, or lose her job. They worry that she will get raped, or pick up AIDS or some other sexually transmitted disease. They worry that she will ruin her health with alcohol and drugs, or end up in jail. They worry that the family reputation will suffer.

HOW BAD IS IT?

Whether consciously or not, most of us apply much stricter standards of behavior to girls and women than to boys and men. Swearing, smoking, drinking, staying out late, skipping school or work, sexual experimentation—all these are considered worse in a female than in a male. But a young woman who defies these conventions may just be *adventurous*. She admires the traditional "male" privileges of independence and mobility, and simply co-opts them for herself.

> *"When I was seventeen, I set out very deliberately to lose my virginity. One night I said to the guy I was with, 'You know, there's really no reason why we shouldn't go to bed together.' He was shocked, and he gave me a big lecture about AIDS and venereal disease. In the end, though, he was very willing to cooperate."*—Lisa B., age 22.

The young female adventurer who lands on her feet may deserve our admiration, not our condemnation. Challenging the traditional female stereotype can be positive if it leads to personal growth and satisfaction. However, some young women get caught in a self-destructive pattern of delinquency and promiscuity. This is an entirely different story; these women need and deserve help. In psychiatry, the general term for this pattern of out-of-control anger, hostility, delinquency, and promiscuity is *conduct disorder*.

CONDUCT DISORDER: IS IT FOR REAL?

Is conduct disorder a bona fide psychiatric "illness," or is it just a convenient label for any adolescent's objectionable behavior? For many psychiatrists, the jury is still out. Specialists in depression find that many depressed teenagers, male and female, act angry rather than sad. Other research suggests that conduct disorder in teens is an early manifestation of bipolar disorder (manic-depressive disorder)—an emotional imbalance in which periods of mania (angry and/or "hyper" behavior) alternate with normal behavior, or with periods of sad withdrawal. The same medications that help control the mood swings of adult bipolar disorder sometimes help "conduct-disordered" teenagers feel and act better.

We prefer not to prescribe medication for a young woman whose only diagnosis is conduct disorder. If she has depression or bipolar disorder, medicine may help her feel more in control of her emotions—but it's never the cure. She still needs to learn new patterns for dealing with her life.

Let's look at different types of delinquent behavior to get some perspective.

TRUANT OR UNRELIABLE

A girl who skips school, a woman who may or may not turn up for work, shows the world she can't be trusted. We look for the underlying reason.

Parents may unwittingly allow their daughter to develop a pattern of skipping school. Maybe they indulge her every time she complains of a headache or stomachache, and she gets the idea that school really isn't that important.

When a delinquent young girl is living at home, we work with the parents to help establish tighter control. A parent-child contract can be very useful: by sticking to the rules (going to school every day, turning in assignments on time), the girl avoids negative consequences; if in addition she does specified chores (making her bed, cleaning her room), she earns privileges.

The most common cause of erratic, irresponsible behavior is alcohol and drug abuse. Sooner or later, the young woman who skips days of work without giving notice loses her job. If she understands this intellectually, and yet continues to show up only when she feels like it, we look for signs of substance abuse.

"GROWNUP" VICES

The teenage girl who drinks and smokes is striving to achieve an adult image: she's not a baby, she knows how to smoke without choking, she can hold her liquor and even drink others under the table, and so on. Health issues are not high on her list of concerns.

It's hard to impress an adolescent with dire predictions about her health, so we usually work with parents to lay down house rules about smoking and drinking. We also work with parents to help them see that they cannot control every area of a teenager's life. They cannot realistically prevent her from smoking, for example, when she is away from home—but they can make "no smoking" a house rule. As with truancy problems, the parent contract is a good tool.

DEFYING AUTHORITY

It's healthy to question authority, but there are right ways and wrong ways to go about it. The delinquent young woman has not learned how to make her challenges effective. She mostly succeeds in shooting herself in the foot.

The girl who screams, "Shut your mouth, you lousy bitch!" to her teacher may or may not have a legitimate gripe, but she definitely has a counterproductive way of expressing dissatisfaction. Likewise, the woman who turns up in traffic court and tells the judge to go to hell will not succeed in making her ticket disappear.

Defiant behavior often involves communication problems. At the hospital, our unruly girl and women patients use role-playing exercises to direct verbal abuse at one another to help them understand how the verbally abused person feels. Then we help the "abusers" think of ways to express the same complaints without arousing hostility.

OUT ALL NIGHT

It may be appropriate for a grown woman to spend all or most of the night out, but it's never appropriate for a teenage girl.

Parents may hesitate to impose a strict curfew on their adolescent daughter, but we find that a girl is usually grateful when her curfew is spelled out for her. If nothing else, it gives her an excuse not to have sex with a boy who may be putting pressure on her.

As long as the girl is living under her parents' roof, they have a right to demand that she live by their rules. But to keep the system from being all punishment and no reward, they also need to offer enticements toward good behavior. Part of our job is helping parents figure out what they want their daughter to do. When they give her a structure for earning rewards (i.e., free time with friends) as well as avoiding punishment, everyone is happier.

SHOPLIFTING

Shoplifting means getting something for nothing. Often a young woman shoplifts because she thinks she isn't getting certain things she feels entitled to.

Slipping store merchandise into a pocket or purse may be an adolescent prank—the thrill of getting away with something. But we suspect it's often a covert way of evening the score.

Obviously, the shoplifter must be made to stop stealing. At Jefferson, we have used an exercise in which a patient sets up an imaginary business, from raising the start-up capital to waiting on customers. Then one of us takes a walk through the imaginary store, describing what objects we are shoplifting and where we are concealing them. Usually the patient is surprised to find herself feeling resentment and hostility. For the first time, she identifies emotionally with the "wronged" party.

A MATTER OF TASTE

"Delinquent" young women often dress in a way that mocks the current fashions. There's usually nothing wrong with that.

How a person dresses, her style, makes a personal

statement. We don't worry if a woman chooses to dress iconoclastically; this is a harmless and potentially healthy way for her to thumb her nose at the dictates of the fashion industry. Sexually provocative attire, however, may give a message that she does not want to have to live up to.

Sometimes a patient wants to work in a traditional business, but has no idea how to dress for it. Her therapist can help her analyze the conventions of women's business wear so she can "dress for success" if she chooses to.

We do worry when a woman patient fails to keep herself reasonably clean, because this may mean deep depression, psychosis, or advanced drug dependency. In our experience, patients who begin to feel better always start paying more attention to personal hygiene and grooming.

"NOTHING" WITHOUT A GUY

When a girl reaches her mid- to late teens, particularly if she feels she still has no strong personal identity, she may look to a boyfriend for that identity.

To some extent, this is normal behavior: all of us derive a large part of our identity from the reactions of the people around us. But when a girl thinks she's nobody if she is not attached to a boy at all times, she is in an extremely vulnerable position.

When talking with a delinquent or "conduct-disordered" young woman, we pay attention to the important relationships in her life. If she is caught in destructive dependency, we try to help her move toward personal autonomy and dignity. As she gains self-respect, she discovers that she is able to deflect or avoid abuse. Often she abandons the relationship entirely, and feels good about it even though she is temporarily alone. She's likely to find valuable emotional reinforcement in a women's support group.

UNINTENTIONAL PREGNANCY

Delinquency in girls often includes sexual adventures that lead to unwanted pregnancy. In many instances, the reason is not ignorance but deep-seated ambivalence.

The teenage birth rate in America has soared in the second half of this century. In 1950 there were 3.2 million births to unmarried women; by 1986, the rate was up to 9.4 million.

Drawbacks to Contraception

- When you use a contraceptive, you have to admit to yourself that you are sexually active. Many women would rather not admit that.
- Diaphragms, contraceptive foam, condoms—these cut down on the spontaneity of sex. The guy might not like it.
- It's embarrassing to walk into a drugstore, pick out a contraceptive, and then face the cashier.
- Using contraceptive pills means you're always "available" for sex. This makes it hard to say no when you're not in the mood.
- Getting a prescription for the pill, or a fitting for a diaphragm, means the expense and delay of a visit to a doctor.
- Some women get blood clots in their legs, and other potentially fatal medical conditions, from using the pill.

Benefits of Pregnancy

- Pregnancy proves that you are able to have children. This knowledge comes as a relief to many women.
- Pregnancy "proves your womanhood."
- Pregnancy proves you are a valuable person who can contribute something tangible (i.e., a child) to society.
- A baby will love you unconditionally and will always be "cute".
- Pregnancy may push your relationship with a man to its next logical step. For instance, if you're living together, the pregnancy may make marriage seem natural.

With contraceptives legal and easily available, why are there so many unwanted pregnancies? One theory holds that most women are fairly ignorant about contraceptives. Another theory says young women have unconscious motives for getting pregnant: they want to get even with their parents, or trap a man into marriage. A more recent theory suggests that women deliberately take risks with contraception, just as people take risks by not fastening their car seat belts.

According to the risk theory, the woman who "doesn't want to get pregnant" realizes that both contraception and pregnancy have drawbacks as well as benefits. Each time she has intercourse, she does a quick mental cost/benefit analysis, and often concludes that the drawbacks of contraception outweigh the (presumably slight) risk of pregnancy. Eventually, of course, she is likely to get pregnant.

Sex and Disease

After birth-control pills became popular in the 1960s, women's exposure to sexually-transmitted diseases increased dramatically. today, the woman who has several male sexual partners (or just one infected partner), and who doesn't habitually use a spermicide, is at risk for any or all of the following:

- AIDS: A devastating breakdown of the body's immune function, AIDS is almost universally fatal. To date there is no cure.
- Chlamydia: Sometimes symptomless in its early stages, untreated chlamydia may cause pelvic inflammatory disease and, eventually, sterility.
- Genital Warts: These are painless raised bumps on the vulva, vagina, and cervix. The warts start small, but may grow as large as 4 inches across. If infected, they have a bad odor.
- Gonorrhea: Capable of infecting and irritating the genitals, liver, and throat, gonorrhea causes skin rashes and sometimes arthritis.
- Herpes: A viral disease of the genitalia, herpes causes sores that may be painful and that tend to recur.
- Syphilis: After causing one or a few genital sores, syphilis may go silent before re-emerging as a rash and swollen glands. If still untreated, it goes underground again until many years later, when it destroys bones, organs, nerves, or the main blood vessel of the heart.
- Trichomoniasis: this infection, caused by a protozoon, causes vaginal discharge, itching, and possible damage to the cervix.

We work with our patients to help them develop greater autonomy. A woman who knows she has the power to make decisions and choices gains a sense of responsibility about contraception. She also becomes more acutely aware of the dangers of AIDS and other sexually transmitted diseases, and of the need to practice "safe sex."

SEX AS A COMMODITY

What about prostitution? Is the girl or woman who trades sexual favors for money or drugs morally corrupt, or is she a victim of an unjust society?

The adolescent girl who prostitutes herself is often a runaway from an unhappy family. Once her money runs out, she finds that her survival options are extremely limited. Drug dealing, pornography, and prostitution surface as highly paid alternatives to starvation. If she was sexually abused as a child, she will probably be a pushover for the pimp who wants to exploit her.

Much of our work with delinquent young women involves helping them become economically self-sufficient. The greater their ability to earn a decent living, the less their attraction to prostitution.

Sometimes a patient defends her right to switch sex partners frequently and/or to trade sex for money, jewelry, and other goods. Rather than dwell on the philosophical issues, we try to impress upon her the very real dangers of promiscuity and prostitution (AIDS first and foremost, but also syphilis, gonorrhea, chlamydia, herpes, and other sexually transmitted diseases, not to mention physical abuse).

The sexual exploitation of women is enormous, multi-faceted, and largely automatic in our culture.

Movies, soap operas, and TV shows like *Dallas* still shamelessly celebrate the stereotypes of the strong, competent man versus the weak, dumb woman, and the use of sex to gain one's goals. At the hospital, we can't hope to undo all this mischief by ourselves. But we do work with social service agencies, shelters for adolescent runaways, safehouses for battered women, drug and alcohol rehabilitation programs, and support groups to help women gain control over their bodies and, ultimately, their lives.

6

Getting High: Alcohol and Drug Pitfalls

One in every 10 to 15 Americans is a problem drinker, some six million smoke marijuana every day, and more than 25 million have taken cocaine at least once. Abuse of alcohol, illegal drugs, and/or prescription medicines such as tranquilizers is a major public health problem. Where do women fit into this picture?

PART ONE: SLIDING DOWN A SLIPPERY SLOPE

Alcohol is big business. Beer advertisements are a mainstay of baseball and football events. Wine is promoted as the elegant accompaniment to food. Whiskey, rum, and vodka seem to be indispensable props to the elegant lifestyle.

Those most influenced by this kind of publicity are teenagers, who are anxious to prove they are sophisticated. Since alcohol, although legal, is a drug, drinking paves the way for later experimenting with illegal or prescription drugs.

When and Why

When and why does a girl begin to experiment with alcohol? The when part is easy: kids usually drink at parties, and parties may start at age 12 or even younger. The older the teens, the more likely it is that they are experienced drinkers: 92 percent of all high school seniors acknowledge having tried alcohol.

Why is a complex issue. Women who started drinking in their teens give the following reasons:

- *Drinking is exciting.* Because drinking under the age of 21 is illegal in most states, it's fun for kids to take the risks of getting and using alcohol.
- *Drinking is "cool."* If you know how to drink, you're not a baby any more.
- *Everybody drinks.* Drinking is expected behavior at a party. Someone who refuses to drink doesn't fit in.
- *Drinking feels good.* Alcohol loosens up social and sexual inhibitions. Girl-boy relations seem less awkward. Everybody has a good time.

The Gateway Effect

Alcohol is a drug. Ethanol, the active ingredient in any alcoholic beverage, is a central nervous system depressant, something like a sleeping pill. At a high enough dosage, it is also an anesthetic.

The young woman who starts to drink at parties soon gets used to swallowing something to achieve euphoria. If nothing bad seems to happen, it's only a small step to try another method of getting high. Smoking marijuana is typically the next step.

Teens usually think the high from alcohol or marijuana is "soft" and harmless. If a young woman is ready for more of an adventure, she may branch out. There are two main tracks: illegal drugs, including cocaine, hallucinogens such as LSD, designer drugs such as Ecstasy, amphetamine, and heroin; and unauthorized use of prescription drugs, including stimulants, tranquilizers, and sleeping pills. She may try any or all of these.

For most women, drinking becomes just a social grace, and experimentation with illegal and/or prescription drugs is either a brief phase in growing up or an occasional pastime. However, for some women, drinking leads to alcoholism and drug-taking leads to drug dependency. A chronically depressed or anxious woman may drink or take drugs to feel better: this self-medication can be the beginning of addiction. Many of the women admitted to our hospital have emotional troubles *and* an alcohol or drug problem. We place them in a special dual diagnosis program, where they get help for both.

Stages of Abuse

Chemical dependency progresses through four stages:

- *Stage One is experimentation:* trying out alcohol and/or different kinds of drugs to see what happens.
- *Stage Two is seeking* a chemically induced mood swing. Once she knows what a high feels like, she actively pursues it.
- *Stage Three is preoccupation* with the mood

swing. At this point, she plans her day around getting high.
• *Stage Four is needing alcohol or drugs to function.* The fun has disappeared. Now she needs alcohol or drugs just to feel normal.

Of course, no one plans to become dependent on alcohol or drugs. No one wants to believe that chemicals can control her. Teens in particular are apt to have an "it can't happen to me" attitude; in psychiatry we call this magical thinking.

Consequences

A woman's chemical dependency, whether it involves alcohol, drugs, or a combination, affects her health, her family, her job, and sometimes her legal status.

Health and psychological problems may include accidents, lung damage from smoking drugs, nose damage from "snorting" drugs, either obesity or emaciation, liver damage, stomach bleeding, lowered resistance to infection, brain damage, panic attacks, low self-esteem, guilt that depresses or enrages her, secretiveness and loneliness, sexual misadventures, accidental drug overdoses, and suicide attempts.

Personal and family problems may include chaotic finances, child abuse or neglect, social isolation, marital conflicts leading to abuse or abandonment, and separation or divorce.

Job problems include lateness, absences, "on-the-job absenteeism," poor job performance, conflicts with co-workers or clients, and decreased ability to be a team player. If she is criticized she may quit her job in anger. She may be fired, or at least passed over for a raise.

Legal problems include falling behind on bills, taxes, and rent or mortgage payments; arrests for driving while intoxicated; losing her driver's license; arrests for possession, use, and/or sale of illegal drugs; and having her children taken from her.

Special Issues

One of the most serious pitfalls for a woman with a chemical dependency is loss of control over her sexual life:

1 Her need for drugs can lead her to depend on a man who supplies her with drugs or money, whether husband, boyfriend, or pimp. He may then take advantage of her sexually.
2 While she is intoxicated, she pays no attention to contraception or "safe sex." Later on, she may not remember who she was with or what they did together. She's at risk for accidental pregnancy and sexually transmitted disease.
3 If she gets pregnant, her continuing intoxication can harm the fetus. Hospitals in large cities grapple daily with the problem of "cocaine babies," "crack babies," newborns with fetal alcohol syndrome, and infants with AIDS. Some pregnant drug-users have been jailed to prevent further harm to the fetus; others have been sued for "fetus abuse."

PART TWO: CODEPENDENCY, THE CAROUSEL OF DENIAL

Codependency is a condition in which people unwittingly encourage dysfunctional persons to depend on them. It is commonly seen in drug or alcohol addicted families, but can also occur in other settings: "addiction" to gambling or religious piety, chronic illness, or a very rigid, controlled home life. Although codependency isn't just a woman's problem, there *are* more women codependents, for two reasons:

First, more men than women are alcoholics and drug addicts. Their wives and girlfriends add up to legions of codependents.

Second, codependency is a "natural" for women because it involves focusing on others rather than on oneself. It includes:

- Feeling responsible for everything that goes wrong.
- Needing to manipulate people and events so they don't "get out of control."
- Being wrapped up in other people's problems, while neglecting one's own.
- Caring very deeply about others, while forgetting to care at all about oneself.

Of course, codependency differs according to the woman's relationship to the addict. Let's look at the codependent woman in three possible roles: wife, daughter, and mother.

The Codependent Wife

She may have married him because, unconsciously, she found him "familiar"—that is, just like her alcoholic father. Many wives of addicts are also daughters of addicts.

Her biggest problem is that she denies he is an alcoholic or a drug abuser. She doesn't want to believe he has the same problem as her father. Anyway, she assumes there's no way to confront his alcohol or drug problem head-on. She hopes that by minimizing it she can make it disappear.

At the hospital, our first goal is to help her see that he does have a problem, and that ignoring or minimizing it will not make it go away.

Another problem: she instinctively covers up for him whenever he's drunk or high. She tells the boss he has the flu. She tells the bank the payment is in the mail. Why? Because she's afraid—afraid he'll lose his job, or get mad and maybe leave her.

We show her that covering up prolongs his illness by letting him get away with intoxication. Usually she's terrified to step back and let him fall on his face, but that's what she needs to do.

The codependent wife is superwoman. She knows how to cook, clean, shop, do the laundry, look after the kids, choose school schedules, apply for scholarships, type term papers, entertain, write to relatives, mow the lawn, fix a leaky toilet, install a new shelf, wallpaper the hallway, pay the bills, take care of taxes, handle the creditors, *and* work at a full-time job—while he knows how to watch TV and get high.

She needs to find time for herself and her own interests. She may not have given a thought to herself in years.

She is usually reluctant to leave him, even if he neglects or abuses her and the children. The family finances may be a mess: if he goes, perhaps she and the children will have no place to live. Even if she is the family breadwinner, she may feel she isn't "strong enough to make it" without him. She also feels that without a man she is nothing; and because she feels responsible for everything—including making her marriage work—she sees leaving him as an admission of her failure.

We provide vocational counseling to help women gain independence from chemically dependent husbands who are abusive, financially irresponsible, or both. We also work to build up the self-esteem of the codependent wife. Only when she's feeling sure of herself can she find the strength to give him an ultimatum: go for treatment or get out!

She feels trapped and defeated because she is caught in a circular pattern. He gets drunk and wrecks the car, or blows his paycheck on cocaine, or loses his job once again. She criticizes him, he blows up. She threatens to leave. He promises to do better, begs her to stay, tells her how much he *needs* her—and she finds this irresistible. She forgives him, and life goes back to normal...until he slips up again.

We help her see she has choices she never dreamed of. She can earn her own money, put it in her own bank account, develop her own credit history, and pursue her own interests. She begins to see that life has a wide horizon and that she has options.

The Codependent Daughter

She may be a young child, depressed and withdrawn. Or a teenager, defiant and rebellious. Or a young woman, fearful and mistrustful. She is the daughter of an alcoholic or an addict.

Growing up in the care of a chemically dependent parent means living with inconsistency, disappointment, and confusion. The daughter lives in a state of chronic watchfulness. She never knows when she will find Mom pie-eyed, or when Dad will stagger in the front door and collapse in the hall. She fears the shouts and thuds from her parents' bedroom at night. If she jokes and laughs, she may get praise or punishment—she's never sure which. She dreads public scenes; she remembers the school concert where her father got into a fight with the music teacher.

If the alcoholic or addict is her mother, the girl grows up mistrusting and perhaps loathing the very person who was physically closest to her in her childhood. She finds her own womanhood, and particularly motherhood, hard to accept.

If the alcoholic or addict is her father, she may grow up fearful and mistrustful of men. Yet since she loves her father despite his shortcomings, she may unconsciously choose another addict as her husband. Daughters of alcoholic or drug-abusing men face two particular risks: sexual molestation and physical (including sexual) abuse.

An intoxicated father may go after his daughter with sexual games and petting. Besides locking the girl and her father into an unwholesome alliance against her mother, this also colors her feelings about sex. She wants attention from Daddy, but not that way. Yet the attention and the sexual fondling are inseparable: a package deal. This leaves her feeling trapped and hopeless.

The patient whose father sexually molested her needs to untangle the threads of her emotional life. To her, sex was something imposed on her. She needs to learn to express her own emotions, both nonsexual and sexual, through touch.

Some alcoholic or addicted men get violent when intoxicated, and beat or rape their wife and children. The abused daughter may develop borderline personality disorder, which involves extreme, unwholesome dependency, or multiple personality disorder, the classic "split personality" syndrome made famous in films like *The Three Faces of Eve* and *Sybil*. She may run away from home, turning to prostitution for survival. Or she may marry early as an escape. In either case, she's likely to end up dependent on a man who abuses her. A wife whose husband has abused her physically or sexually may develop post-traumatic stress disorder, a nerve-wracking disintegration of her normal coping abilities.

A codependent daughter often has difficulty developing a separate and mature relationship with her parents. She may still feel the need to "take care of" one parent—physically, financially, or emotionally—to the detriment of her own marriage or children.

For women in abusive relationships, vocational counseling and individual therapy help foster self-reliance and self-respect. These women respond enthusiastically to expressive therapy, which gives them an outlet for emotions they have had to suppress all their lives.

The Codependent Mother

When a teenager abuses alcohol or drugs, the mother usually has a hard time recognizing the evidence. Her blindness comes from love, and a desperate wish to preserve her integrity as a parent; surely only the child of a bad mother would abuse alcohol or drugs! She makes excuses for outrageous behavior: he failed his course because he didn't get along with the teacher; he wrecked the car because he misjudged the curve.

We gently unveil her child's pattern of abuse, and help her see how she has been kidding herself and "sweeping dirt under the carpet." She is incredulous, then angry, then afraid. Finally she wants to make changes within the family to help ensure that her child will stay sober and/or straight.

The problem is that teenagers are moving naturally toward independence from their parents. When a teen returns home from an alcohol and drug rehabilitation program, however, his parents need to exert tight control until he can prove he deserves their trust. The most useful tool for this purpose is the family contract: a list of "house rules" and a method for earning extra privileges (phone time, time with friends) through good behavior.

The "Cure" for Codependency

The codependent woman wants above all else to be loved—by her husband, her child, her parent, whoever. Even if she disagrees with someone, she can't afford to take a firm stand for fear of losing his love. She goes along with what he wants, even if it's something destructive. Her only self-esteem comes from other people's praise for what she can do for them.

She needs to learn to love herself first—this will be her key to self-esteem and healthy relationships. Building self-esteem is the core of therapy for codependency.

7

Fat Phobia: The World of Eating Disorders

"The thinner you are, the prettier you'll be." In America, thin equals attractive—and not just to adults. Preschool girls virtuously sip diet cola along with their portion of birthday cake. By age 5 they already understand that thin is in.

The pressure increases as these girls grow older. A survey of American high school girls showed that 70 percent were dissatisfied with their bodies and wanted to lose weight. In another survey, 80 percent of high school senior girls wanted to lose weight: 30 percent were dieting at the time, and 60 percent had dieted earlier in the school year.

Ads, movies, and TV shows all scream that thin means desirable. The rewards for a thin body are said to include popularity, fulfilling sex, a wonderful marriage, and high self-esteem. The perfect body is supposedly achievable; all you need is a little willpower and some money. Women spend their time and earnings on diet powders and all kinds of cosmetic surgery: breast enlargement or reduction, tummy tucks, face lifts, liposuction.

IS FAT A DISEASE?

Most doctors consider obesity a disease. Overweight is said to contribute to heart disease, high blood pressure, diabetes, arthritis, and gallstones. Regardless of their medical history, overweight people are supposed to get tough with themselves and slim down.

(Interestingly, research suggests that overweight is not always correlated with heart attack. What precipitates heart attack in overweight people may sometimes be the stress of repeated dieting! Being underweight may be more of a health risk than being slightly, and stably, overweight.)

If a diet doesn't do the trick, some doctors may suggest a hospital-supervised fast, or even surgery—cutting away fat tissue, removing a portion of the intestines, stapling the stomach or filling it up with a balloon.

Surgery is by no means a foolproof way to lose weight, and it can be dangerous. After an intestine-shortening operation a woman may have diarrhea for weeks or months, and/or increased susceptibility to arthritis and gallstones—two of the conditions that weight loss is supposed to cure! Surgery for obesity is *fatal* up to 10 percent of the time.

BULIMIA: THE FEAST-AND-PURGE CYCLE

Hundreds of diet books promise quick, easy, guaranteed weight loss ("Shed 17 pounds the first week!")

Women's magazines reprint these diets, sandwiched between ads for luscious high-calorie foods and drinks. TV also juxtaposes ads for diet drinks with ads for candy. The message: Women should make and buy goodies, but not eat or drink them. "Buy! Eat! Enjoy!" but also "Avoid! Limit! Ration!"

For some women, the conflicting urges to eat and be slim coalesce into bulimia or bulimarexia: binge eating, then purging through vomiting or laxatives. At first it seems ideal—eating a lot without suffering any caloric consequences. There are emotional rewards, too: binge eating relieves tension; vomiting involves muscle spasms that can come to feel stimulating; purging causes a temporary "high." By the time the drawbacks appear, bulimia has become an obsession—a pattern that keeps running automatically. It's hard to know how many women have bulimia; one survey of college women found that 4 to 7 percent of them binged and purged to some extent.

Mountains of Treats

The woman with bulimia favors soft, rich foods that go down fast. She may eat up to 40,000 calories a day in multiple binges, yet get rid of all the food before her body has a chance to absorb it. One bulimic who weighed only 62 pounds spent a full six hours a night eating.

Buying, hiding, eating, and then purging huge amounts of food requires privacy, so the woman with bulimia becomes secretive. She plans her day around her secret binges. One bulimic bought shopping carts full of cookies every day, explaining to the checkout clerk that she was a nursery school teacher buying snacks for the kids. Because her food habit was expensive, she stole whatever she could. She hid her purging from her family by vomiting in a bathroom that had a very loud ventilator fan.

Criteria for Bulimia

Bulimia involves the following:

- Recurrent binge eating: rapid intake of very large amounts of food.
- Hiding the binge from other people.
- Ending the binge when other people show up, or when stomach pain develops.
- Finishing a binge by vomiting or falling asleep.
- Repeatedly going on severe diets, and "helping" the diet with vomiting, diuretics, or laxatives.
- Bounding between high and low weights (more than 10 pounds' difference) because of fasts and binges.
- Feeling depressed after a binge.
- Knowing that binges and purges are harmful, but being unable to stop.

Continued purging does serious harm to the woman's body. Stomach acids from vomiting wear away her tooth enamel and make her gums recede. Acid and abrasion erode her esophagus, causing bleeding (and in some cases, fatal rupture). Purging depletes her body of potassium and other minerals, damaging the nervous system and making her vulnerable to convulsions, slow or irregular heartbeat, and low blood pressure.

The woman with bulimia may need nutritional supplements. She also needs therapy to help her build self-esteem, express her emotions, and relax. When she explores the spiritual side of her personality— whether through formal religion or individual meditation—she may find a calm that she needs and values.

A planned program of physical exercise is an ideal tool for recovery. However, obsessively exercising "to burn off calories" can be one more trap for the bulimic woman. At the hospital, we design our therapy program to keep the exercise level moderate.

ANOREXIA NERVOSA: OVERCONTROL

For one in every 250 young women, concern about gaining weight develops into the disorder called anorexia nervosa: compulsive dieting that turns into self-starvation. The most common age for the onset of anorexia is between 13 and 22 years, although girls as young as 11 and women up to age 60 have become anorectic.

The teen who goes on a diet hopes to achieve an "ideal" appearance, plus feelings of greater control over her eating and her weight. If she is happy and comfortable in her relationships with family and friends, she may succeed without harming herself. But if she is lonely and uncomfortable with other people, her diet may end up taking over her life. She may use dieting as a weapon:

- *Defensively,* to ward off what she perceives as other people's disapproval of her fatness; and/or
- *Offensively,* to capture the secret prize of being the thinnest one of all.

Criteria for Anorexia

Anorexia involves some or all of the following:

- loss of 20 percent of normal weight
- cessation of menstruation
- dry skin
- constipation
- thinning of hair on the head
- new growth of downy body hair called lanugo
- low body temperature (as low as 95 degrees)
- low blood pressure (i.e., 80/50)
- slow pulse rate (as low as 39 beats per minute)
- abnormally low levels of potassium and chloride in the blood (if she vomits frequently)

The anorectic young woman starves herself relentlessly. She has not lost her appetite—in fact, she is hungry all the time—but her obsession with thinness makes her shun food. She may abuse diuretics and laxatives in addition to dieting, and she exercises fanatically. Her perception of her body becomes distorted; even when she has reached skeletal thinness, she thinks she sees fat that still needs to be dieted away.

The woman with anorexia is performing a mental trick: simplifying all her concerns about popularity, self-worth, and lovability into a single overriding concern about fatness. Anorexia is her attempt to conquer fears and insecurities by gaining absolute control in one area: body weight. Once she organizes the game of life this way, it seems simple. If she loses weight, she wins. If she puts on weight, she loses.

Naturally, her obsessive dieting eventually leads to severe malnutrition. If it continues too long, it may not be reversible: 10 to 15 percent of anorectic women die of their disorder. It's crucial to get a woman with anorexia to treatment right away. The longer anorexia continues, the harder it is to overcome. At the hospital, we can closely monitor our anorectic patients' blood pressure, pulse, respiration, heartbeat, and edema (tissue swelling). Regular blood tests are used to check for levels of calcium, magnesium, potassium, and chloride.

If a recovering woman gains weight too fast, she is prone to heart failure. This is one reason why the woman with anorexia needs close medical supervision, as well as therapy based on understanding and trust rather than forced feeding.

Relatives May Make Things Worse

Family members may unwittingly make things worse. Often they too are overly concerned with weight; their message may be, "Eat, but don't get fat." If they cheerfully tell the anorectic patient she's "looking good," she may take this to mean she looks fatter—just what she fears! They need to learn that her weight loss and peculiar eating habits are not the problem, but symptoms of her problems in managing her life. We find that effective treatment for an eating disorder must include extensive family therapy, as well as individual counseling.

THE "EATING DISORDER" PERSONALITY

Whether she has bulimia or anorexia, the woman

with an eating disorder is also struggling with certain life issues. Characteristically these include:

- *Perfectionism.* To feel worthy, she thinks she needs to be perfect in every way: perfect (i.e., thin) body, perfect thoughts, perfect grades, perfect housekeeping.
- *Low Self-Esteem.* Since she is striving for an unattainable "perfect body," failure is guaranteed. The recurring failure undermines her sense of self-worth.
- *Dependency.* She feels inadequate, and wants to lean heavily on something or someone who takes away her feeling of helplessness.
- *Struggle for Power.* If other people try to make her stop dieting, she fights them using intimidation, manipulation, and guilt.
- *Sexual Identity Questions.* Is her body thin enough to please a man? Why should she please a man, anyway? If she stops having periods and loses all her curves, can she avoid sexuality altogether?
- *Secrecy.* She knows her dieting is self-destructive, but since her sense of control depends on it, she hides it. Secretiveness makes her lonely.
- *Depression.* A biological depression may have caused the feelings of worthlessness that made her focus obsessively on her weight.

Because of these life issues, treatment for women with eating disorders must be comprehensive. The woman needs to deal not only with her harmful habits of starving or gorging-and-purging, but also with her idea of herself and who she wants to be.

WHAT ABOUT THE CONSTANT DIETER?

What about the woman who is neither bulimic nor anorexic, but whose life is one unending diet? Although she is unlikely to seek therapy for an eating disorder, her preoccupation with food and body weight is psychologically crippling. It is definitely a "minus" rather than a "plus" in her life.

At Jefferson, our Women's Program group therapy sessions include discussion about food and body image, even for patients who don't have eating disorders. We encourage women to step off the treadmill of compulsive dieting and calorie-counting.

A woman can free herself from slavery to "fat phobia" by developing an independent personal identity. With the support of other women, she can free herself from those powerful cultural demands for thinness.

To women who feel they are overly wrapped up in fears about fatness, we propose the following goals:

1 Accept the fact that you are a complex person. Don't simplify everything to a question of fat or thin, good or bad.

2 Learn how to reach out to others for help. You can't solve all your problems by yourself.

3 Become a flexible decision-maker. Learn how to change your plans quickly when things don't work out as expected.

4 Dare to trust yourself. This will allow you to trust others, too.

WHAT IS HUNGER?

Women who hate themselves for being overweight should think and talk about what they really feel when they are "hungry." Insight into "hunger" can help dissolve the compulsion to eat all the time. Here are some reasons why a woman might eat compulsively:

Food is a reward. A mother may promise her child a cookie for good behavior. It's easy to adopt the habit of rewarding oneself frequently with a sweet snack.

Food is a consolation. Often life metes out unexpected "punishments." A hot fudge sundae can seem soothing.

Food is a legitimate treat. Many women hesitate to spend money on clothes or entertainment for themselves—but food is okay because it's a necessity of life.

Food is a celebration. Food plays a key role in festivities—birthday, anniversary, wedding, promotion, raise, graduation.

Food fosters sociability. Maybe she isn't the least bit hungry, but she sits down and eats because dinner is a time for family togetherness.

Food is a pastime. When she's bored and doesn't know what else to do, she eats to fill the time.

Food calms and soothes. While some women can't eat when they are nervous, others find that food gives them a lift.

Food wards off future hunger. She may think she's eating now so she won't "die of starvation" later.

We advise the woman who is unhappy about her

compulsive eating to eat only when she is actually hungry. Since she has probably lost her ability to tell what real hunger is, we ask her to follow a three-step approach:

1 Pay attention to when and how she eats, to learn what "hunger" means to her.
2 Go without food for a number of hours, so real hunger has a chance to develop.
3 Slowly and thoughtfully eat only enough to satisfy her real hunger.

The compulsive eater's big task is to revise her relationship with food. When she learns to distinguish between her need for nourishment and her needs for consolation, stimulation, reward, and reassurance, she will gradually break free from her compulsion. We encourage good nutrition that includes all the food groups in a varied diet. We also believe in moderate exercise—with others, having fun!

FOOD AS A SYMBOL

Because food ensures survival, it exerts a powerful influence on people's minds. It's easy to let food become a symbol. The anorectic woman lets food symbolize fatness, repulsiveness, and rejection. The bulimic woman sees food as something extremely desirable, but forbidden. And the compulsive eater grabs at food as if it were life's ultimate, but elusive, reward.

For many women today, coming to terms with food—seeing it for what it is, and not as a symbol for something else—is one of the major tasks of growing into adulthood.

8

Motherhood:
Blessing or Curse?

Some of our patients are mothers, and wish they weren't. Others are not mothers, and wish they were. Some who have chosen to be full-time mothers come under fire for neglecting their careers; others who have chosen to be childless are scorned or pitied for missing out on life. Is being a mother a blessing, a curse, or a little of both?

In our experience, motherhood and the potential for motherhood are extremely emotional issues. They loom so large in the psychological development and the psychiatric treatment of women that we have decided to devote a whole chapter to them.

A GIRL'S PERSPECTIVE

As a growing girl gradually realizes that she may someday have children, she mentally runs through various scenarios: One child, or several? Daughters, sons, or both? A city apartment, or a house in the suburbs? A husband who changes diapers, or not? Grandparents who are doting, or distant?

When she starts to menstruate and knows that this means the beginning of fertility, the issue of motherhood suddenly takes on added seriousness. If a boy shows an interest in her, she may scrutinize him in terms of fatherhood potential.

As she becomes sexually active, she encounters new dilemmas. If she grows up in a traditional middle-class home, she learns that pregnancy before marriage would be a social disgrace. She shelves the idea of motherhood for the time being, and concentrates on other things: social life, studies, career plans.

CHOICE OF LIFESTYLE

Girls who assume they will someday have children eye their mothers, teachers, and other women for clues about how motherhood fits into the rest of a woman's life. By her early twenties, assuming she has not yet had a child, the woman perceives a number of life-plan options for herself. Author Gail Sheehy, in her book *Passages,* describes these options. Briefly, they are:

- *Caregiver.* The woman centers her life around her husband and their home. What matters is creating and maintaining a warm, welcoming, nurturing environment for the two of them and, before too long, their children.
- *Either-Or.* Caregiving and career seem equally important, but mutually exclusive. Either she goes for nurturing and caregiving first, postponing achievement until after her children are grown; or she achieves first, postponing moth-

erhood and caregiving until she's settled in a career.

- *Integrator.* Caregiving and career do *not* seem mutually exclusive; she goes for both of them at the same time. After a day on the job, she rushes back home to be nurturing.
- *Deliberately Childless.* She embarks on a career with no thought of making time later for children. Mothering is not necessarily repugnant to her; it's just foreign to the way she leads her life.
- *Transient.* Not knowing "what she wants to be when she grows up," she decides to experience as much as possible. She may travel a lot, change jobs often, and experiment with different lifestyles. Eventually, she will probably choose one of the above options.

Thus, a woman's life plans always involve a decision, or at least the postponement of a decision, about becoming a mother.

CONCEPTION AS A CHOICE

For much of history, a woman had little choice about conceiving a child. Once she was married, she was expected to have children as soon as nature saw fit to arrange it. Not all women had children, of course: some couldn't, some never married, and some joined a religious order that practiced celibacy. But the woman who married gave her implicit consent to becoming a mother sooner or later. "Birth control," until recently, was a male prerogative.

Naturally, women were not always thrilled to find themselves pregnant. Those who felt they absolutely must not give birth—because they were not married, were in poor health, or already had more children than they could care for—tried desperately to abort. They took whatever measures they could think of, or consulted clandestine specialists. In the Middle Ages, "witches" purportedly knew how to induce abortion. The Christian church opposed abortion. In the U.S. there were no laws against abortion initially. These were later introduced to protect women, particularly against back-street abortionists. In the United States, it wasn't till 1973 that the Supreme Court's *Roe v. Wade* decision affirmed a woman's right to choose abortion. Currently that right is being challenged by laws severely restricting abortion in some states.

A MOTHER'S JOB

Bearing children, though hazardous enough in the days when many women died of post-childbirth bleeding or infection, was only the beginning. For centuries, the household was a self-contained unit that bound family members together in a logical interdependence. Since foods, clothing, and medicines did not come from factories, the housewife's work was vital to everyone's survival. In addition to preparing meals, preserving food, and making clothing, the mother was in complete charge of the children—assigning their chores, and teaching them to count, read the Bible, and write. Many women made money "on the side": raising chickens and selling the eggs, taking in laundry or sewing for the well-to-do. The children often worked, too!

Today, technology and social change have lightened women's traditional workload. Clothes and dishes can be washed by machine; diapers are disposable. Fresh foods are available all year round; meal preparation is quicker and easier; few women sew except for fun. Formal education is the schools' responsibility. Most family units no longer "produce" anything; a child's daily chores have dwindled to the level of making her bed or putting her laundry in the hamper.

Today's mother might seem to have little to do. Yet anyone who has ever had a child, or even watched a young mother, knows this is untrue. Babies and young children require constant care and supervision, and these cannot be mechanized. In addition, expectations have changed. A mother's competence is now judged by how many books her children know by heart; how soon they can count, say the alphabet, and name their colors; how well they can talk. It takes time and effort to impart this knowledge. Today's mom is also judged by how her children are dressed; how many museums and nature centers they've visited; how many kinds of cuisine they've sampled; how soon they started learning to play a musical instrument. It takes money to provide these experiences.

If the woman is wholeheartedly committed to being a full-time mother, and if she is married to a wealthy man who provides amply for her and the children, life can be rosy. However, few mothers are so enviably comfortable. Some chafe at having to curtail their professional activities. Others have limited budgets, or are the sole providers for their children.

DRAWN TO OPPOSING GOALS

Many mothers today are caught in a cultural dilemma: how can they reach their own dreams of personal fulfillment, spend years of their life cherishing and nurturing their children, *and* provide the children with all the material goods and educational advantages that define a "wonderful childhood"?

When we look again at those lifestyle options open to young women, we see that each has its deficiencies:

- *Caregiver.* She feels inadequate if she forgoes a career. Not only is she economically weak and vulnerable, but she probably feels limited and "boring."
- *Either-Or.* If she starts to work only after raising a family, she's competing on a job market that's teeming with high-powered career people. At age 45, she may have less prestige and lower earning power than a new college grad.

  If she works and postpones having a family, she worries chronically about whether she's doing the right thing—and whether she'll be able to get pregnant when she wants to.
- *Integrator.* If she pursues a challenging or time-consuming job while rearing young children, she's apt to be physically and psychologically overwhelmed by the demands of both.
- *Deliberately Childless.* Even if *she* has no doubts about her femininity and womanhood, others inevitably do. She has to stand up to various degrees of pity, scorn, and bafflement expressed by relatives and friends.
- *Transient.* If she is traveling and changing jobs frequently, her biggest problems are loneliness and lack of a sense of purpose.

We help our patients see that they should not try to be all things to all people. A woman needs the freedom to choose a lifestyle option and stick with it for as long as it feels right—and then to change options, when she needs to, without guilt.

Advances in contraception mean women have more reproductive freedom than ever before, yet freedom does not necessarily mean happiness. We see conception-related problems in many of our patients:

GETTING PREGNANT

"We had been married about a year when I found out I was pregnant. My first thought was, Oh, no! My parents will kill me!"—Pregnant woman, age 28

"Believe it or not, the first time in my life that I felt totally comfortable with my body was when I got pregnant. Suddenly it was okay to gain weight and let my stomach stick out."—Young mother, age 31.

Contraception Can Fail

Many women live from one month to the next in fear of not getting their menstrual period. As you saw in Chapter Five, knowledge about contraception does not necessarily mean consistent use of contraception. Birth control pills can have side effects, some of them serious. Spermicides can fail. Getting a diaphragm means making, keeping, and paying for a doctor's appointment. Condoms require the male partner's cooperation. Buying contraceptive products can be embarrassing.

The Biological Clock Ticks On

Women who are concentrating on their careers, but want children eventually, grow increasingly aware of the passage of time. They may be depressed and anxious without realizing they are preoccupied with the question of when to get pregnant.

Our Culture Says a Woman Should Be a Mother

It also says she should be a wage-earner. She may find herself unhappy no matter which option she chooses. Guilt and self-doubt can cripple her in whatever type of work she has chosen.

Pregnancy May Feel Like Coercion

Whether the woman got pregnant accidentally or on purpose, nothing short of an abortion can stop it. She may fear or resent the gradual changes in her body. The onslaught of new sensations and perceptions may cause her to panic.

If a woman feels deep conflict about getting pregnant, we try to help her see the issues objectively: Are there goals she deeply wants to reach before having a baby? Is she responding to social pressure rather than to her own desire for a child?

When a pregnant woman is approaching motherhood with trepidation, we help her explore options she may not have thought of: Can she reduce her workload from full-time to part-time? Can someone help her care for the child?

LIFE AS A MOTHER

Once the physical upheaval of childbirth is over, a woman may feel marvelously fulfilled in her new motherhood. Conversely, her new role may be tearing her apart. She may feel at war with her body (will she ever shed those extra pounds?) and with her self-image (is she now good only for hushing a crying baby by shoving a nipple in its mouth?) She'll probably experience both extremes, feeling by turns fulfilled and exasperated.

As time goes on, she will probably find satisfaction in motherhood. Yet, simultaneously, she chafes at the loss of her personal liberty. If she has a daughter, she faces an especially delicate task, because she must prepare the girl for the complications and ambiguities of womanhood. If she feels thwarted in her ambitions to "make something of herself," she may drive her daughter to achieve and stand out. Or she may discourage her from having any ambitions at all.

WHAT IS A MOTHER WORTH?

A homemaker may think she "really doesn't work." But a study done in the 1970s by the Chase Manhattan Bank calculated that a full-time homemaker works 99.6 hours per week at 12 or more jobs (nursemaid, dietician, food buyer, cook, dishwasher, housekeeper, laundress, seamstress, practical nurse, maintenance worker, gardener, and chauffeur) and gets no pension plan and no health, medical, or accident insurance. When state and private employment agencies were asked to fill a job of that description, the response was disbelief and amusement.

What is the solution? Should mothers be paid for staying home to look after children and keep house? Should every employer be required to provide on-site day care?

Many of the problems of supervising children are actually social issues. It makes no sense that a woman who works should fear for her children's welfare and safety during after-school hours, or on days or weeks when the children are not in school. Likewise, it's absurd that a woman with half-grown children be the only one in her family to cook, clean, and do laundry.

We encourage women to push for day-care facilities, and subsidized after-school and summer programs. We also encourage the wife-and-mother to require that her husband and children do a significant portion of the housework. Often, she must first teach them how!

HOW TO COPE WITH EVERYTHING

Most of all, we teach women the technique of planning their lives in sequences. Rather than expecting to have everything all at once, they can see life as a series of stages, each with its own set of emphases. For example, a woman might work full-time in her chosen field, then have children and do little or no paid work but stay in touch with her field, then go back to work part-time or become a freelancer.

The male model of a career need not be the female model. Few women need or want to be Superwoman. For a mother, the real question may not be how to get out of the house and back into the office as fast as possible, but how to reintegrate paid activity into her life without relinquishing her mothering role.

Motherhood can be rewarding—or frustrating. A career can be exciting—or empty. Trying to combine the two can be fulfilling—or exhausting. There is no "right answer" for everybody. The important thing is to make the choices for oneself, do what feels right at the time, and be prepared to change if feelings or circumstances change. Once a decision is made, it has to be accepted without regret, but with the flexibility to make future changes. One can always change the future, but never the past. Accepting this is the basis for serenity.

9

Fear Moves In: Anxiety, Panic, and Phobias

In the condition called agoraphobia, being in a public situation causes anxiety or panic. By reputation it's a "woman's problem," and in fact two-thirds of agoraphobics are women. Why? Is a woman's biochemistry more vulnerable to agoraphobia than a man's? Are women culturally more susceptible?

There are other, related questions. Why do more women have panic and anxiety disorders, and compulsive cleaning or "avoiding" rituals? What's going on here, and what can be done about it?

WHAT IS ANXIETY?

Anxiety is basically fear that arises from nowhere. Ordinary fear is an understandable reaction—to an earthquake, let's say, or a near-accident—but pathological anxiety is an irrational fear of a remote, unlikely danger. The anxious person senses that something terrible is about to happen. Since she does not know what it will be, she fears many things, depending on where she is and what's happening.

For example, if she worries constantly about her child's safety, during the course of a day she may fear that he will be hit by a car on the way to school, get head lice from the other children, injure himself in gym, ruin his eyes playing a video game, set the house on fire while making himself popcorn, develop a vitamin deficiency from refusing his vegetables at dinner, fall out of bed at night, and so on.

Or she may be worry about what will happen to herself. She may live in dread of losing control: vomiting, fainting, perhaps even dying. She is constantly irritable and on edge.

Common Physical Signs of Anxiety

lightheadedness	stomach discomfort
sweating	lump in the throat
cold hands	high pulse rate
dry mouth	rapid breathing
racing heart	numbness in hands or
urinary urgency	feet
diarrhea	frequent sighing
trembling	pallor
jumpiness	flushing
inability to relax	

WHAT IS PANIC?

Panic is very intense anxiety. When it overcomes the person suddenly and without warning, it's spontaneous panic. When worry about an upcoming situation escalates into trembling, rapid heartbeat, sweating, and a fear of loss of control, this is anticipatory panic. If the symptoms are less severe, they are called spontaneous or anticipatory anxiety.

During a panic attack, the sufferer is short of breath and feels heart palpitations, a choking sensation, chest pain, dizziness, trembling, and faintness. She may be afraid she is going crazy or dying. Intense panic usually abates after half an hour or less (whereas anxiety may last for hours, days, or even weeks at a time). Panic is sometimes part of agoraphobia; the person suffers a panic attack when she is in an "exposed" situation from which she can't make a quick exit, or she fears she *will* panic in this kind of situation.

WHAT ARE THE ANXIETY DISORDERS?

Anxiety disorders, which may or may not involve panic attacks, include the following:

- *Panic Disorder.* This consists of recurring panic attacks that develop out of the blue. It most commonly starts in late adolescence or early adulthood, and strikes women somewhat more often than men. Panic disorder may disappear after a few attacks, or it may evolve into a crippling long-term problem. In women who suffer from panic disorder, a classic danger is self-medication: overuse of alcohol, or of unauthorized prescription drugs, to dull the discomfort of the attacks.
- *Generalized Anxiety Disorder.* This involves a high level of diffuse fear and anxiety for a month or more, but without panic attacks.

- *Obsessive-Compulsive Disorder.* The person's fixation on certain thoughts (killing someone, running outside naked) or rituals (hand-washing, being neat) is so consuming that it interferes with normal functioning. Women are more apt to get involved in obsessive cleaning and avoiding of "contaminated" objects or situations; men are more apt to develop an obsessive ritual of checking to see that a task (closing the door, turning down the thermostat) has been done right.
- *Obsessions.* These are unwanted, intrusive thoughts that seem to take over the person's mind. They may be about violating social or moral taboos, or they may have a religious theme.

WHAT IS A PHOBIA?

Phobia is an irrational fear of something that is not objectively threatening and that most people are not afraid of. Fear of air travel is quite common, for example: 10 percent of people refuse to take a plane at all, and 20 percent have considerable anxiety or even panic if they do fly. People have phobias about animals, spiders, insects, closed spaces, thunder, heights, and so on.

Agoraphobia is by far the most common of the phobic disorders. An agoraphobic may fear church, restaurants, highway driving, doctor's appointments, theaters, escalators—any place where there are crowds or where she might not be able to retreat quickly.

In some women, a panic attack signals the start of agoraphobia; in others, panic attacks start only after agoraphobia has developed. Fear of having a

---

Different Types of Phobias

Agoraphobia: Fear of being trapped in a (usually public) situation.

Claustrophobia: Fear of suffocation in an enclosed place.

Social phobia: Fear of being humiliated in a social situation.

Social skills deficits: Extreme shyness; inability to make friends.

Dysmorphophobia: Delusion that a part of one's body is disgusting.

Specific phobias: Dread of one or several objects or situations: pointed objects, spiders, travel, flying.

Illness phobia: Fear of catching a particular disease, such as cancer or tuberculosis.

Blood-injury phobia: Fainting or feeling faint at the sight or mention of blood, an injury, or a needle.

---

panic attack can keep a woman literally housebound. Women who have relatives suffering from depression, an anxiety disorder, or alcoholism seem especially vulnerable to agoraphobia.

WHAT IS POST-TRAUMATIC STRESS DISORDER?

After a sudden, violent physical or emotional shock, or repeated traumas such as physical or sexual abuse, a person may suffer from incapacitating flashbacks, nightmares, anxiety, and depression. This set of symptoms, which is called post-traumatic stress disorder, may clear up within six months or so—or it may last for years. The person may function poorly in all aspects of her life, or only in certain specific areas.

Many of the studies of post-traumatic stress disorder have involved male soldiers who experienced violent combat. Yet women can and do suffer from this condition. Female victims of rape or violent crime may be deeply and permanently affected by their ordeal. Other women who develop post-traumatic stress disorder include victims of crashes, kidnapping or torture, fires, cave-ins, or natural disasters; and witnesses of disasters, including families and friends of the victims, firefighters, police officers, and rescue workers.

IS THERE SUCH A THING AS AN "ANXIOUS PERSONALITY?"

Scientists have never been able to pinpoint an "anxiety-prone personality." People who suffer from anxiety and/or panic do share certain characteristics: they tend to have low self-esteem, be prone to guilt feelings, daydream often, have a low curiosity level, and shrink from new sensations. However, it's unclear whether these characteristics are the cause of anxiety or the result of it.

A more fruitful area of investigation is physical illness; several physical disorders can produce feelings of anxiety or even panic. Among them are:

- *Heart conditions,* including angina, heart attack, abnormal heart rhythms, congestive heart failure, and very low blood pressure.
- *Lung problems,* such as emphysema and asthma.
- *Brain and nerve disorders,* including epilepsy and vertigo.

• *Hormone and glandular conditions,* such as underactive thyroid, overactive thyroid, and diabetes.

An adverse reaction to a drug or medication can sometimes cause anxiety. Too much caffeine makes many people jittery. Alcohol is another culprit (both heavy drinking and withdrawal from drinking). Various street drugs occasionally produce intense anxiety. Medications known to cause anxiety in some people include stimulants, diet pills, cold remedies, antispasmodics, digitalis, some blood pressure medications, and sleeping pills. Paradoxically, even antidepressants, which may be prescribed to help overcome panic, may cause anxiety in some people. A woman who has been taking a tranquilizer such as Xanax or Valium may experience anxiety attacks when she stops taking the pills, especially if she stops suddenly instead of tapering off.

THEORIES ABOUT CAUSE: A WOMAN'S PERSPECTIVE

Physical illness-related or drug-related anxiety aside, we don't really know what causes most cases of anxiety and panic. There are a number of theories, however, each of which has particular nuances regarding women patients.

The psychodynamic theory. This says anxiety results from unconscious conflicts over unpleasant childhood experiences: discomfort, abuse, or sexual trauma. Unfortunately, unearthing hidden conflicts does not usually erase anxiety or panic states. The assumption that parents—and in particular, mothers—cause their children's unconscious conflicts makes for a great deal of unnecessary guilt.

The learning theory. This says that when a person feels nervous in a situation, she learns to avoid it, and eventually develops a pattern of fear and avoidance. The learning theory makes sense, since deliberate, repeated exposure to the feared situation or object can help many people overcome their fears.

The genetic theory. This says anxiety-proneness is an inherited characteristic. Scientific evidence does support a genetic connection: identical twins with anxiety disorders, for example, tend to have the same fear at the same level of intensity. A single genetic factor may cause several related disorders: within a given family, for example, the men may tend toward alcoholism and the women toward agoraphobia or depression.

The developmental theory. This says human beings are "programmed" with certain inborn fears that may once have had survival value. There's considerable evidence that the following fears are at least partly innate: fear of heights, fear of being stared at, fear of strangers, fear of dead or mutilated bodies, fear of darkness, fear of a dark forest, fear of snakes, and fear of novelty.

The biochemical theory. This says that an imbalance in a person's body chemistry causes anxiety attacks, and that correcting the imbalance will dissolve the anxiety. Body chemistry does change in response to stress, sometimes making the person more vulnerable to anxiety attacks. Interestingly, medication is not the only way to "fix" a biochemical imbalance: counseling and behavioral therapy may also induce biochemical changes.

SO, ARE WOMEN MORE VULNERABLE THAN MEN?

As you have seen, women are definitely the majority of agoraphobics, but men take the lead in certain obsessive-compulsive types of behavior. Thus, overall, women are no more likely than men to suffer from an anxiety state. Women and men suffer in equal numbers from these seeming short-circuits in the psychobiological wiring.

Is stress, then, the cause of anxiety disorders? Certainly, most people who suffer from anxiety overreact to the stresses in their lives, and often a person with a phobia can remember a stressful event that seemed to trigger her irrational fear. However, even though all of us are exposed to stresses throughout our lives, most of us do not suffer from anxiety disorders.

For whatever reason, people are intrinsically different from one another. Exposing three people to the same stress is like hitting three bells—one plastic, one glass, one metal—with a hammer: the plastic dents, the glass shatters, and the metal rings. Certain people are particularly vulnerable to the development of incapacitating anxiety. The reason may be the genes they inherited, their early childhood experiences, their daily diet, their work environment, the air they breathe—or a combination of some or all of these. Gender roles—those "parts in the play of life" that society doles out, some to women and others to men—partly determine who suffers from which anxiety disorder.

WHAT HELP IS AVAILABLE?

Fortunately, a great deal of help is available for women with anxiety disorders or phobias. The approach we favor has five components: behavior therapy; medication if appropriate; psychotherapy; support therapy; and exercise.

- *Behavior therapy* teaches the patient how to face and tolerate the object or situation that frightens her. With enough exposure, her fear will diminish to a manageable level, and eventually disappear altogether. Post-traumatic stress disorder, in particular, can be arrested if the person is taken back early and often to the scene of the trauma.

- *Medication* is not a panacea, but it may give therapy a definite boost. For anxiety states and panic attacks, the right medicine may be Inderal, a beta-blocker; Tofranil or Prozac, antidepressants; or Klonopin, Valium or Xanax, tranquilizers. Many phobias abate in response to Benadryl, an antihistamine, or Dramamine, an antinausea medication. Some obsessions and compulsions disappear in response to Prozac, a relatively new antidepressant. Anafranil is a new medication which specifically reduces obsessions and compulsions.

- *Psychotherapy,* or talk therapy, is most effective in treating anxiety disorders when it concentrates on the here-and-now as well as on what might have happened in infancy or childhood. Helping the patient understand the dynamics of her personal relationships can help her change those relationships in ways that satisfy her. Teaching her to understand her feelings, dreams, and daydreams can likewise help her make constructive changes. The therapist can suggest new, positive ways of thinking to replace the old, self-defeating patterns.

- *Support therapy* can mean empathy and reassurance from the individual therapist, chicken soup from family members, and/or sharing of experiences in a support group. Because the families of patients also need support and guidance, we at Jefferson Hospital schedule special family sessions. Often, a patient who has been the only caregiver in her family finds it touching when her husband and children start giving help and support.

- *Exercise* is a good therapeutic tool. Women, in particular, are often too narrowly focused on how they look and out of touch with how they feel physically. Regular exercise lifts mood and reduces anxiety. We encourage women to become more physical beings as they work their way out of anxieties, compulsions, and phobias. Most of them find joy in this new outlet for their energies.

10

Gloom Takes Over: Depression and Suicide

Both women and men suffer from depressive illnesses. Yet in the United States, depression is *the* leading psychiatric diagnosis for women. Overall, depression is twice as common in women as in men; in the 25- to 44-year-old age group it is three times as common in women. What do these figures mean?

- One theory is that women are quicker to seek help; that is, a lot of depressed men just don't get counted. There may be some truth to this.
- A second theory is that women are emotionally weaker, and thus more prone to depression. We doubt this is true. In fact, we are continually impressed by women's emotional resilience.
- A third theory is that doctors are counting wrong. Since depressed men often turn to alcohol, their diagnosis is likely to be alcoholism, not depression. This is also likely to be true, particularly since family studies have shown

an association between females diagnosed with depression and males diagnosed with alcoholism.

- A fourth theory is that life is more complex for a woman: when she feels she can no longer cope, she's ripe for depression. To us, this has the ring of truth. Many women, in their struggle for physical and psychological health, must deal with incredible stress.

RECOGNIZING DEPRESSION

All of us have had "down" days when we felt too negative to do anything useful or fun—but then the mood lifted and we felt normal again. To understand depression, imagine that, instead of lifting, the gloom stretched out indefinitely... and deepened.

To the person with clinical depression, day follows dreary day and nothing seems to get better. Even though there may have been no obvious event that triggered the depression, her waking hours are filled with sadness, flatness, and boredom, or possibly anguish, anxiety, and restlessness. Food seems tasteless; friends and family seem remote. Getting to sleep at night, or staying asleep, is a problem. The future looks bleak. Thoughts revolve around the past, and there is a pervasive sense of guilt. Life seems stupid and pointless.

A depressed person may think she is suffering from some incurable disease that no one will tell her about. She may believe very sincerely that the end of the world is imminent. She may hear "voices" that blame her for some unspeakable wrongdoing. These are examples of delusional thinking, which is sometimes, but not always, a part of severe depression.

In unipolar depression, the person becomes depressed, stays depressed for some time (weeks or months, depending on how soon and how effectively she is treated), eventually emerges from the depression, and functions normally again.

Characteristics of Depression

- extreme tiredness or fatigue
- decreased level of activity
- feeling of boredom with usual activities and pastimes
- loss of interest in sexual expression
- inability to think and concentrate normally
- lack of appetite (or sometimes food cravings, surprisingly big appetite, and weight gain)
- trouble falling asleep or staying asleep
- exaggerated feelings of guilt and worthlessness
- thoughts of harming or killing oneself
- impaired job or school functioning
- increased irritability

There is, however, a second basic type of depression. It is actually the depressive phase of bipolar illness (also called manic-depressive illness). In bipolar illness, the person has one or more episodes of unnaturally excited, "hyper" behavior, either before or after one or more episodes of depression. When she is depressed, she appears to have "regular," unipolar depression. Yet she probably will get little or no benefit from the medications that help people with unipolar depression. She needs a different type of medication. One that works well for many patients is a salt of the metal called lithium.

RECOGNIZING MANIC STATES

People with manic-depressive illness experience, at least once, several days or weeks of a supercharged emotional state. If it's nothing more than exuberance, sleeplessness, fast talking, and excessive activity, it's called *hypomania* (sub-mania). If it escalates into an uncomfortable "speedy" feeling, recklessness, dangerous risk-taking, delusions of omnipotence or of persecution, and irritable, angry reactions to others, it's called *mania*. A person who has at least one bout of hypomania or mania, and at least one period of clinical depression, may be diagnosed as having bipolar disorder.

MISUNDERSTANDINGS ABOUT MANIC-DEPRESSIVE ILLNESS

One very common myth is that mania and depression always take equal turns. Actually, in many patients, the depression of manic-depressive disorder can be difficult to distinguish from "regular" de-

---

Characteristics of Mania

- a sustained euphoric or irritable mood
- unusually high level of activity and sociability
- persistent state of sexual arousal
- thoughts that seem to race through the head
- unpleasant feeling of mental and physical speeding (and perhaps the desire for alcohol or tranquilizers in order to calm down)
- hurried, pressured way of talking
- tendency to spend and give extravagantly, far beyond one's means
- little or no need for sleep

pression. A woman who once had a manic episode might go on to have several bouts of depression with no intervening mania. If she seeks treatment for depression, but does not volunteer the information that she once suffered from mania, the doctor may prescribe an inappropriate medication—one which might help lift "ordinary" depression, but which probably will not relieve the manic-depressive type of depression.

Is "Conduct Disorder" Really Bipolar Disorder

According to recent thinking, at least some delinquent youngsters may have a bipolar disorder. In a girl, classic signs of "conduct disorder" are lying, truancy, running away from home, and self-destructive promiscuity. A boy with conduct disorder may additionally set fires, break into houses or cars, destroy property, act cruelly toward people and animals, commit muggings or purse-snatchings, force sex on others, start physical fights, and fight with weapons. All this is remarkably similar to adult "manic-depressive" behavior.

Another common myth is that bipolar disorder is exclusively an adult's illness. Increasingly, psychiatry is realizing that bipolar disorder often starts in adolescence. Each year, thousands of delinquent, obstreperous teenagers are diagnosed as having "conduct disorder." Many of these poorly behaved young people may in fact be showing early symptoms of bipolar disorder.

WHAT'S BEHIND SUICIDE?

Many depressed people think seriously of suicide, and in the United States some 300,000 to 400,000 a year attempt to kill themselves. Suicide is the ultimate act of despair: the person feels unworthy of living, and *acts* on that feeling. In spite of herself she may see every knife or razor blade as a tool for opening a vein, every bridge or high building as a potential place to jump from. The risk of suicide makes it imperative to treat severe depression rather than let it run its course.

Strangely, suicide is most apt to occur when the person is beginning to emerge from her depression. While she is most deeply depressed, she is often too incapacitated to take any initiative at all. If she still feels overcome by despair and self-loathing, but suddenly gets back a little of her energy, she may use that energy to end her life. This is why psychiatrists strongly recommend hospitalization for a severely depressed patient.

Fortunately, only 10 percent to 15 percent of all people who attempt suicide succeed in killing themselves. The majority of suicide victims are men, not women: national suicide rates for 1986 were 19 per 100,000 for men, versus 5 per 100,000 for women.

Attempts at suicide are a different story; women account for about two-thirds of all unsuccessful suicide attempts. Partly this is because women are less likely to use guns, which allow for no second thoughts. Instead, women tend to overdose on medications, and are often found in time to be rescued. We think a woman's failed suicide attempt indicates not ineptness, but a reservoir of hope and strength.

IS DEPRESSION PURELY BIOLOGICAL?

Several different kinds of medication can help patients overcome depression. Unipolar depression requires one kind of medication, and the depression of manic-depressive illness requires another kind.

Does this imply that depression is purely a physical illness, and that the cure need be nothing more than a few pills a day? In our opinion, no. Even if medication is highly effective in lifting depression, a depressed patient *also* gets a great deal from reviewing and re-evaluating her life in "talk therapy." Just as unhappy life circumstances can lead to depression, improved conditions can lead out of depression. It's up to the patient, with her therapist, to sort out what the life issues are:

- Extremely difficult survival problems, such as hunger and homelessness, may have precipitated her depression. Medication may help her feel better temporarily, but she will need social and vocational support to help her achieve more strength and self-direction.
- Her depression may center around a destructive relationship. A woman who is abused at home needs to disengage emotionally from the person who abuses her, establish an alternative living arrangement, and rebuild her self-esteem.
- Depression may be a reaction to social norms she feels she can neither live with nor ignore. If she is attracted to other women, for example, but does not dare "come out" as a lesbian, despair and frustration may be at the heart of her depression.
- Depression may also result because a woman has not learned to deal with stress. Instead of expressing her feelings, she has been programmed to "be good."

We believe the ideal treatment for depression or manic-depressive illness is three-pronged: (1) medication, if appropriate, to improve or stabilize mood; (2) counseling to sort out important life issues; and (3) education about the illness—not only for the patient, but also for family members who are struggling to understand what she is going through.

WHEN DEPRESSION STRIKES THE HUSBAND

When a husband is depressed, his spouse may blame herself for not being a good enough wife—and he may encourage her to think that way! Whereas the depressed wife often tries to conceal her feelings of isolation and estrangement, the depressed husband, unaccustomed to blaming himself for anything, may "explain" to his wife that he has fallen out of love with her—or that his unhappiness stems from her shortcomings as a housekeeper, cook, bedmate, or mother.

Or a husband's depression may show up as sudden, inexplicable trouble on the job. Perhaps he gets a much-coveted promotion, only to begin doubting that he really deserves it. If he is in the manic phase of manic-depressive illness, perhaps he alienates the boss by acting loud and obnoxious, or by promising customers more than the company can possibly deliver.

A woman should know that if her husband begins to act in an entirely uncharacteristic way—either elated/angry or subdued/depressed—the blame does not lie with her. He probably needs treatment for a depressive disorder. She should refuse to accept the blame for his emotional state, and she should insist that he get a thorough medical and psychological evaluation.

WHEN IT'S THE CHILD WHO IS DEPRESSED

Children's depression can look quite different from that of grownups. The depressed child may mostly show extreme irritability: screaming, temper tantrums, violent accusations.

In children, as in grownups, severe depression can sometimes cause hallucinations or delusional thinking. Depressed children as young as 5 or 6 have attempted suicide, and some have succeeded. About 5,000 American teenagers a year take their own lives.

Mothers need to know that children can suffer from depression—and that depression in children is treatable. An evaluation by a child psychiatrist is crucial for correct diagnosis and treatment.

For several decades after World War II, "the experts" blamed mothers for everything that went wrong with their children's emotional development. If a little boy became autistic, his mother had not loved him well enough. If a girl had a psychotic break, her mother had not given her a strong sense of identity. If a young woman chose not to marry, her mother had thwarted her psychosexual maturation. If a man had obsessions and compulsions, his mother had toilet-trained him too severely.

Today, the discovery that many emotional illnesses are associated with abnormal biochemical states is gradually reversing the tendency to fix the blame on Mom. We now understand that style of parenting is only one of the factors that shape a child's emotional development. Other important influences include inherited characteristics (depression and bipolar illness seem to run in families), environmental influences (emotional integrity can deteriorate with prolonged malnutrition or exposure to polluted air or water), and cultural variables (racial prejudice warps a

---

Suicidal Adolescents: Warning Signs

Any of the following may be a tipoff that a teenager is at risk for suicide:
- a history of learning disabilities
- a history of physical or sexual abuse
- a history of previous suicide attempt(s)
- alcohol and/or drug abuse
- obviously depressed mood
- very frequent complaints of illness
- increased irritability and problem behavior
- withdrawal from friends
- loss of interest in school
- giving up formerly pleasurable hobbies
- no longer caring about grooming and appearance
- giving away valued possessions
- no longer making plans for the future
- preoccupation with themes of death and dying
- saying, "I wish I were dead"

---

child's developing self-esteem). To be effective, therapy for depression must take into account *all* of these influences.

Mothers and Daughters: Special Tensions

Since mothers teach their daughters about womanhood largely by example, and since the female role in our society is fraught with ambiguity, the mother-daughter relationship in particular tends to be full of unspoken, largely unrecognized tensions. A daughter who is depressed may find her mother a convenient target for her own confusion and frustration about becoming a woman. The girl may openly despise her mother for her fatness (or thinness), criticize her for not having a career (or for having one), hate her for imposing overly strict house rules (or for not imposing any).

A mother whose daughter abuses her, verbally or physically, must put a stop to this—for her own sake and for the sake of her daughter. She needs to work with a competent, compassionate therapist who can correctly diagnose the problem, prescribe any medication that might be needed, and work with her, the daughter, and other family members to establish new guidelines for acceptable behavior.

11

Breaking Out Of the Mold

To sum up, too many women today are still invisible within our culture—locked away inside an old, confining role that's no longer useful to them or their loved ones. Too many are strong, capable, and resourceful but think of themselves as weak, incompetent, and dependent. The right therapy can help a woman break out of the "dependent" mold, take charge of her life, and become more visible—to herself and, eventually, to others.

CRISIS INTERVENTION

Let's start with a worst-case scenario: a woman in physical, mental, or emotional crisis. Maybe she's having panic attacks, and is getting more and more afraid to leave home. Maybe she's strung out on booze and drugs: sick and anxious, missing days of work, wondering where she spent last weekend. Maybe her boyfriend just walked out on her, and she's so distraught that she's thinking of suicide. Maybe her husband just gave her another black eye.

A crisis calls for immediate help. Where should she turn? Ideally, to a place like Jefferson Hospital where there's comprehensive care: medication if necessary, individual counseling, group therapy, expressive therapy, vocational advice, education for her and her family, and follow-up care.

What's Wrong With Good Old Doc?

Can't a woman in difficulty just turn to her family doctor for help? Family doctors, while a precious national resource, may not be the best helpers for women in emotional or mental crisis:

- Most family doctors had only a brief exposure to psychiatry during their medical training. They don't pretend to be experts at diagnosing the problem underlying an emotional or mental crisis.
- Family doctors aren't usually experts at prescribing mood-altering medication. They may prescribe a less-than-ideal medication, or the right medication at the wrong dosage.
- Family doctors don't usually provide the individual counseling that's vital in treating emotional or mental crisis.

When the Crisis Passes

Let's assume the woman gets competent psychiatric help. Within a few weeks, the worst is over. She no longer feels crippled by panic. Or she has achieved a tenuous abstinence from alcohol and drugs. Or thoughts of suicide no longer obsess her. Or she is no longer living with a man who beats her up. After the crisis, however, the real work begins! Now is the time for her to consolidate her psychological gains and develop some perspective.

If her panic attacks are subsiding in response to medication, her task is to boost her own confidence by exposing herself, little by little, to situations that used to make her anxious. If she has managed to stay off alcohol, pills, and drugs for a few weeks, her task is to reinforce that abstinence by going to AA meetings and finding new emotional outlets. If her suicidal depression is gradually lifting, her task is to reach out to other people and rebuild the links that broke when she was isolated in her despair. If she has separated herself physically from an abusive man, her task is to make that separation durable.

Individual counseling can help her develop perspective. As she and her therapist discuss her life, they may find evidence of a family tendency (whether inherited or picked up through example) toward a particular kind of emotional distress. They may discover that she has accepted harmful ideas about "a woman's place." Together, they piece together a picture of her mental and emotional life, and try to decide what caused her crisis.

Holly, for instance, was a feminist who prized her independence. When she began to have panic attacks and to avoid public places, she was not only terrified but baffled and ashamed: was she betraying her own principles? In therapy, she realized that agoraphobia ran through her family: several of her aunts and cousins suffered from the same syndrome. Thus, her panic attacks probably resulted from faulty biochemical "programming"—not some dark wish to attract protective attention. With her self-doubt removed, Holly felt her well-being soar. Medication helped diminish her panic attacks, and she was able to resume her normal, active life.

Joanna, on the other hand, found that her problems stemmed from attitude and circumstance, not biochemistry. Joanna had low self-esteem and few job skills, she had been mired in a violent relationship for seven years. Often she threatened to leave her abusive husband, but she never did it because she depended on him financially. When she first came for treatment, she was suicidally depressed. In counseling, Joanna realized she definitely would leave her husband if she knew she could support herself. This spurred her to enroll in an intensive job training program, which eventually became her ticket to freedom from abuse.

EMOTIONAL VOCABULARY-BUILDING

Another important part of therapy is helping the woman name her repressed feelings. Most of the women we see need practice in identifying and expressing their inner feelings.

As we saw earlier, standard "ladylike" behavior leaves little room for anger. Yet over the course of a lifetime, a woman is bound to have moments of deep anger. Learning how to express her anger prevents her from turning it against herself. (Significantly, one definition of depression is "anger turned against oneself.")

Also, typical "ladylike" behavior encourages feelings of inappropriate guilt. These days, guilt is a familiar feeling to many conscientious women, because woman's role seems to be expanding endlessly. It's not enough to be a good wife, housekeeper, and mother, and it's not enough to be a good breadwinner;

today's woman feels she has to be all these things—
and a good cook and entertainer, too, and it helps a lot
if she's thin and dresses like a fashion model! Guilt is
repressed anger, which, as we've seen, causes depression. To let go of guilt, a woman needs to choose which
expectations she really wants to meet.

Often a woman tries to control uncomfortable
feelings by ignoring them. Counseling helps her put a
name to her feelings so she can deal with them.
Anxiety is one of these uncomfortable feelings; fear of
rejection is another. The woman who represses either
or both of them appears hard and uncaring. When she
learns to acknowledge and express her anxieties
about other people, she appears more receptive—and
people respond to her with greater warmth.

The woman who dreads conflict may find herself
inwardly angry that she is always bending over back-
ward to please others. Or she may feel immobilized,
caught between equal forces pulling in opposite directions. In counseling, she discovers that conflict itself is
not bad: what counts is how she handles it. Learning
to spell out the conflict helps her resolve it constructively.

If she swallows her grief when a relationship
ends or a loved one dies, the grief may go underground, only to resurface much later in the form of
severe depression. Grieving over a loss is natural,
appropriate, and necessary for healing.

Sometimes the emotional "vocabulary" is nonver-
bal. That's why we encourage our patients to vent
their anger on a punching bag, or explore their crea-
tivity through drawing, painting, and sculpture. In
addition, women who are expanding their emotional
repertoire find that it helps to concentrate on simple,
long-forgotten pleasures: the beauty of a flower, a
landscape, music, waves on a beach, or people's
voices.

RECOGNIZING HARMFUL STEREOTYPES

One of therapy's vital functions is teaching a woman to recognize the stereotypes that degrade and devalue her. Stereotypes that women at Jefferson have pinpointed and criticized include these:

- *Sex Object.* "Women are put on earth to flatter men and gratify their sexual desires. Women's bodies are suitable for commercial use: they give products an aura of sexuality and seduce consumers into buying."
- *Saint.* "Women are made to give and serve endlessly. They gladly sacrifice *all* their needs, wants, and ambitions to those of men and children."
- *Idiot.* "Women can't think rationally and have no head for figures. Ring-around-the-collar is all they know about chemistry."
- *Victim.* "Women are weak, inept, and helpless; they need men to protect and rescue them."
- *Castrator.* "Women try to enslave their husbands and sons. Mothers who are too powerful make their children neurotic or even psychotic."
- *Enemy to Other Women.* "Women are cruel, petty, slyly competitive, and constantly out to steal other women's husbands or boyfriends."

Once a woman recognizes the limitations these stereotypes impose, she can create her own definitions of who and what she is.

DREAMING NEW DREAMS

Another goal of comprehensive therapy is to help

a woman recognize and articulate her hidden dreams. In many cases, a woman assumes her dreams will never come true because she is powerless to direct the course of her life. One of our greatest pleasures is watching a woman discover that she *can* shape her future: that her dreams can become reality.

Since college days, Barbara's highest achievement had been her ability to "drink anyone under the table" at parties. In her mid-forties, her alcoholism finally cost her her husband, her children, and her job. Hospitalized for detoxification and rehabilitation, she learned to abstain from alcohol, one day at a time. But the heartwarming part of the story came later, when Barbara found that her knack for making ornamental wreaths and wall ornaments had commercial value. With advice from a friend, she started a business; within 18 months she was a successful entrepreneur. Barbara was not just "cured" of her alcoholism. She now had a public persona; she had become visible.

Ann was not born in the United States. She came here after she met and married her husband, who was in the U.S. Navy. She had been sexually abused by her father, but had repressed this memory due to her feelings of shame. As an adult she was depressed. Although she loved her children, she easily became enraged when they weren't "perfect."

In therapy she began to realize that this was because her identity was wrapped up in being a good mother—if the children misbehaved, she felt inadequate. She wanted to get a job, but because of her inadequate education she could only work as a kitchen helper, which she found very frustrating. Through therapy she learned how feelings of guilt and inadequacy had sapped her self-confidence. She decided to enroll in a GED course, and eventually obtained a degree in social work—a goal which she could not have dreamed of when she first came to see us.

Ellen, who'd had phobias and anxiety attacks since childhood, was so socially handicapped that she had barely managed to graduate from college. She led a homebound existence, occupying herself with housework, prayer, and Bible reading. When her husband became disabled and their finances deteriorated, she began clerking in a department store, but panic attacks made her miss so much work that the store let her go. At this point, she came to Jefferson. Thanks to a combination of medication, behavior therapy, and counseling, she was able to take a job again within several months. But the best was yet to come: With her new-found confidence, Ellen began to feel a deep calling to the ordained ministry. She applied to a seminary, got a scholarship, became a doctor of divinity, and now leads an urban parish.

EVOLVING SEXUALLY

Most of the patients in the Women's Program find that their sexuality evolves and matures as they take control of other aspects of their lives. All-female group therapy lets them discuss sexuality freely—in some cases, for the first time in their lives. A woman who shares her personal history of sexual molestation or abuse often unwittingly acts as a catalyst; her story may trigger other women's repressed memories of sexual trauma or discomfort. As they talk over their experiences, they realize that their sexuality exists by itself, not just as a response to a man's wishes. In group discussions about sexuality, some of the sexual myths that women expose are these:

- A woman's genitals are dirty and disgusting, but a man's are clean and beautiful.
- Sex is dirty and shameful for women, but clean and healthy for men.
- If a woman doesn't feel like being sexual when a man wants her to, she's frigid.
- If she feels like being sexual when he doesn't want to, she's a nymphomaniac.
- Having sex means being penetrated by a man's penis; anything else is either "foreplay" or "afterplay."
- There's only one right way to have an orgasm; man on top and active, woman underneath and passive.
- If a woman doesn't have an orgasm every time she has intercourse, something's wrong with her.
- Masturbation is a last-resort form of sexuality.
- Handicapped people have no sexual feelings.

Debunking these sexual myths, and replacing them with real information, frees women to experience their own bodies.

As a woman expands her mental horizons, she sees that sexuality can be much more than genital activity. Jogging until she reaches a "runner's high," soaking in a perfumed bath, pulling on a luxurious silk slip, moving to the beat of rhythmic music—all are sensual feelings, whether she's alone or with someone. The woman who pushes herself to unlearn negative stereotypes usually discovers many new pleasures. As her own sexuality becomes more visible and available to her, she acquires a stronger sense of presence.

GROWING POLITICALLY

Women grow more radical as they get older. As a woman looks back, she sees that many of her past troubles stemmed from social and cultural prejudices against women. She learns new ways to root for woman as the underdog: thumbing her nose at fashion, ignoring sexist jokes, spurning organizations that exclude women, treating other women with respect regardless of their social class. A woman who is taking control of her life usually acquires some political visibility. She first needs to find out what public issues are important to women's lives. Some examples:

- *Reproductive Freedom.* As this book goes to press, ultraconservative Americans are trying to persuade the Supreme Court to take back women's right to choose abortion. Also, a French "morning-after" pill that could eliminate the need for many early abortions, and which has several other medical uses, is being kept off the U.S. market for political reasons.
- *Drug Testing.* For hormonal and other reasons, women may react to medications quite differently from men. So far, however, pharmaceutical companies are not required to test a new drug's effect on women before they release it for sale.
- *Health Insurance.* As of 1990, the United States and South Africa were the only two "developed" nations that did not guarantee *all* their citizens access to basic medical services. In America, many unemployed people, part-time employees, and low-paid workers who do not qualify for Medicaid—including millions of women and their children—can't afford health care.

- *Child care*. Although child care is the underpinning of a mother's ability to hold a paid job, child care centers are relatively scarce and expensive. Only a few businesses offer or subsidize child care as an employee benefit. What's needed is a grassroots political effort to make good, affordable child care available to all families who need it.

Keeping informed, writing and talking to her elected officials, making contributions, organizing, demonstrating: all give a woman political power. All increase her visibility—to herself, and to others who look to her for inspiration.

WOMEN CHANGING PSYCHIATRY

For too long, mainstream psychiatry has minimized women's issues. It's up to all of us to see that this changes. If you're a woman and you need psychiatric care, make sure your therapist supports your need for autonomy, strength, and dignity—make sure she enhances your visibility! You'll be doing yourself, and everyone else, a priceless favor.

Sources

Burt, Pauline, and O'Brien, Patricia H.: *Stopping Rape.* New York, Pergamon Press, 1985.

Beattie, Melody: *Codependent No More.* New York, Harper & Row and Hazelden Foundation, 1987.

Boston Women's Health Collective: *The New Our Bodies, Ourselves.* New York, Simon and Schuster, 1984.

Braiker, Harriet B.: *Getting Up When You're Feeling Down.* New York, Putnam, 1988.

Campbell, Bebe Moore: *Successful Women, Angry Men.* New York, Random House, 1986.

Cardozo, Arlene: *Sequencing.* New York, Atheneum, 1986.

Chesler, Phyllis: *Women and Madness.* San Diego, New York, and London, Harcourt Brace Jovanovich, 1972 and 1989.

———and Goodman, Emily Jane: *Women, Money, and Power.* New York, William Morrow and Co., 1976.

Chodorow, Nancy J.: *Feminism and Psychoanalytic Theory*. New Haven and London, Yale University Press, 1989.

Doress, Paula Brown, Siegal, Diana Laskin, and The Midlife and Older Women Book Project: *Ourselves, Growing Older*. New York, Simon and Schuster, 1987.

Ehrenreich, Barbara, and English, Deirdre: *For Her Own Good*. New York, Anchor Press/Doubleday, 1978.

Extein, Irl; Herridge, Peter, and Kirstein, Larry: *New Medicines of the Mind*. New York, Berkeley Books, 1989.

Evans, Glen, and Farberow, Norman L.: *Encyclopedia of Suicide*. New York, Facts On File, 1988.

Friday, Nancy: *My Mother, Myself*. New York, Dell Publishing Co., 1977.

Gilbert, Sandra M., and Gubar, Susan, editors: *The Norton Anthology of Literature By Women*. New York, W. W. Norton, 1985.

Gold, Mark S.: *The Good News About Depression*. New York, Bantam Books, 1987.

———: *The Good News About Panic, Anxiety & Phobias*. New York, Villard, 1989.

Goodwin, Donald W.: *Anxiety*. New York and Oxford, Oxford University Press, 1986.

Gornick, Vivian, and Moran, Barbara K.: *Women in Sexist Society*. New York, Basic Books, 1971.

Greist, John H.; Jefferson, James W., and Marks, Isaac M.: *Anxiety and Its Treatment*. Washington, D.C., American Psychiatric Press, 1986.

Hall, Lindsey, and Cohn, Leigh: *Bulimia: A Guide to Recovery*. Carlsbad, Calif., Gurze Books, 1988.

Hendricks, Lorraine: *Kids Who Do/Kids Who Don't*. Summit, N.J., PIA Press, 1989.

Hyde, Janet Shibley: *Half the Human Experience.* Lexington, Mass., D.C. Heath and Co., 1985.

Ketcham, Katherine, and Mueller, L. Ann: *Eating Right to Live Sober.* New York, New American Library, 1986.

Kinoy, Barbara P., et al: *When Will We Laugh Again?* New York, Columbia University Press, 1984.

Klein, Donald F., and Wender, Paul H.: *Do You Have a Depressive Illness?* New York, New American Library, 1988.

Lerner, Harriet Goldhor: *The Dance of Anger.* New York, Harper & Row, 1985.

Levenkron, Steven: *Treating and Overcoming Anorexia Nervosa.* New York, Warner Books, 1982.

Levinson, Harold N.: *Phobia Free.* New York, M. Evans and Co., 1986.

Levitt, Eugene: *The Psychology of Anxiety.* Indianapolis, Bobbs-Merrill Co., 1967.

Linedecker, Clifford L.: *Children in Chains.* New York, Everest House, 1981.

Lips, Hilary M., and Colwill, Nina Lee: *The Psychology of Sex Differences.* Englewood Cliffs, N.J., Prentice-Hall, 1978.

Macdonald, Donald Ian: *Drugs, Drinking and Adolescents.* Chicago, Year Book Medical Publishers, 1984.

McDonnell, Kathleen: *Adverse Effects.* Ontario, International Organization for Consumers Unions and The Women's Press, (co-publishers), 1986.

Miller, Jean Baker: *Toward a New Psychology of Women.* Boston, Beacon Press, 1976.

Mitchell, Juliet: *Psychoanalysis and Feminism.* New York, Random House, 1974.

Morgan, Elaine: *The Descent of Woman.* New York, Stein and Day, 1972.

Orbach, Susie: *Fat Is a Feminist Issue*. New York, Berkeley, 1978.

————: *Hunger Strike*. New York, Norton, 1986.

Papolos, Demitri F., and Papolos, Janice: *Overcoming Depression*. New York, Harper & Row, 1987.

Pearson, Carol S.: *The Hero Within*. San Francisco, Harper & Row, 1986.

Rapoport, Judith L.: *The Boy Who Couldn't Stop Washing*. New York, E. P. Dutton, 1989.

Rothenbert, Paula S.: *Racism and Sexism*. New York, St. Martin's, 1988.

Sanford, Linda Tschirhart, and Donovan, Mary Ellen: *Women and Self-Esteem*. New York, Anchor Press/ Doubleday, 1984.

Sheehy, Gail: *Passages*. New York, E. P. Dutton, 1974.

Slaby, Andrew E.: *Aftershock*. New York, PIA Specialty Press, 1989.

Sobel, Suzanne Barbara, and Russo, Nancy Felipe, editors: *Professional Psychology, Special Issue*. Arlington, Va., American Psychological Association, 1981.

Wegscheider, Sharon: *Another Chance*. Palo Alto, Calif., Science and Behavior Books, Inc., 1981.

Wilson, R. Reid: *Don't Panic*. New York, Harper & Row, 1986.

Index

A

Abortion
  historic perspective, 85
  political issues, 123
Abuse. *See* Physical abuse;
    Psychological abuse; Sexual abuse
Acquired immune deficiency syndrome (AIDS), 57
Adolescence
  chemical dependency, 51
  codependent daughters, 67-69
  delinquent behavior, 50-59
  depression, 111-113
  pregnancy, 55-58
  psychiatric patterns, 44
  social crises, 42-44
  substance abuse, 60-64
  suicidal signs, 112
Aggression, in women, 33
Agoraphobia, 92, 96, 116-117
  panic with, 94, 95-96
AIDS. *See* Acquired immune

deficiency syndrome (AIDS)
Alcohol
  barbiturates and, 23
  children of alcoholic parents, 67-69
  gateway effect, 61-62
  media contribution to use, 60
  teenage use, 51, 60-61
  treatment for alcoholism, 116
  when experimentation begins, 61
  why people drink, 61
Anafranil, 101
Androgyny, 15
Anger
  freedom to express, 12, 117
  in women, 33
Anorexia nervosa
  age group effected, 75
  control issue, 76
  family role, 77

ABOUT THE AUTHORS

Dr. Joyce Stapp attended Indiana University for formal training. She completed her residency in psychiatry at the University of Louisville in Louisville, Kentucky. Presently, Dr. Stapp is the medical director for the Women's Program of the Adult Services at Jefferson Hospital in Jeffersonville, Indiana. She specializes in treating codependent adult and adolescent survivors of physically, sexually, and emotionally abusive homes.

Dr. Beryl Langley grew up in England and attended King's College Medical School of London University. After spending two years working in the pediatric field in Jamaica, she came to the United States to pursue further training in psychiatry at the University of Missouri, and in child psychiatry at Washington University in St. Louis. She was in private practice in Virginia for several years before moving to Louisville, Kentucky to become Medical Director of Jefferson Hospital. Dr. Langley is board certified in psychiatry, and is a member of the American Psychiatric Association, the Academy of Child and Adolescent Psychiatry, the American Medical Women's Association and the Association of Women Psychiatrists.